Pocket Guide to
Cultural Assessment

Pocket Guide to
Cultural Assessment

ELAINE M. GEISSLER, PhD, RN, CTN
Tolland, Connecticut

Illustrated

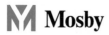

Mosby

St. Louis Baltimore Boston Chicago London Madrid
Philadelphia Sydney Toronto

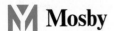
Mosby

Dedicated to Publishing Excellence

Executive Editor: Linda L. Duncan
Developmental Editor: Kathy Sartori
Project Manager: Patricia Tannian
Production Editor: Barbara Jeanne Wilson
Senior Book Designer: Gail Morey Hudson
Cover Designer: Teresa Breckwoldt
Manufacturing Supervisor: Betty Richmond

Special Recognition: Maps reprinted from *The Software Toolworks World Atlas* with permission. Copyright 1989-1993, Electromap Inc., Fayetteville, Arkansas. (All Rights Reserved)

Printed in the United States of America
Composition by Graphic World, Inc.
Printing/binding by R.R. Donnelley & Sons Company

Mosby–Year Book, Inc.
11830 Westline Industrial Drive, St. Louis, Missouri 63146

Library of Congress Cataloging in Publication Data

Geissler, Elaine Marie.
    Pocket guide to cultural assessment / Elaine M. Geissler.
        p.   cm.
    ISBN 0-8016-6752-6
    1. Transcultural nursing—Handbooks, manuals, etc.   I. Title.
RT86.54.G45   1993
610.73—dc20   93-28745
                                                                    CIP

95   96   97   /   9   8   7   6   5   4   3

ANNA AWLASEWICZ, RN, BS

Student, School of Nursing, University of Connecticut
Storrs, Connecticut

Romania

INGALENA BERGH, RN, BSc

Head of Planning
Stockholm College of Health and Caring Sciences
Stockholm, Sweden

Sweden

BARBARA J. BROWN, RN, EdD, FAAN

Associate Executive Director of Nursing
King Faisal Specialist Hospital and Research Centre
Riyadh, Saudi Arabia, 1987-1991

Saudi Arabia

CARMEN-ROSA CHILICKI, RN, BS

Student, School of Nursing, University of Connecticut
Storrs, Connecticut

Poland

MARGA COLER, RN, CS, CTN, EdD

Professor of Nursing, University of Connecticut
Storrs, Connecticut

Brazil

ØYVIND DAHL, PhD

Associate Professor, Center for Intercultural Communication
Stavanger, Norway

Madagascar, Norway

TOMMY DAHLEN, PhD

Student, Department of Social Anthropology
Stockholm, Sweden

Sweden

LINDA DUNCAN, RN, BS

Student, School of Nursing, University of Connecticut
Storrs, Connecticut

China

BETTE GEBRIAN-MAGLOIRE, RN, MPH, PhD
Haitian Health Foundation
Jeremie, Haiti
Haiti

ELEANOR KROHN HERRMANN, RN, EdD, FAAN
Professor of Nursing, University of Connecticut
Storrs, Connecticut
Belize

JAMES R. KURTZ, RN, MPH
Primary Health Care Consultant, Ministry of Health
Lao PDR
Laos

CAROLYN LANGER, RN, MS
Student, University of Connecticut
Storrs, Connecticut
South Korea

NURGUN PLATIN, RN, DNSc
Associate Professor, Chairperson of Pediatric Nursing
Hacettepe University, Ankara, Turkey
Turkey

HANS-JOACHIM RIEKE
Berlin, Germany, Participant, 1991
Summer Institute for Intercultural Communication
Portland, Oregon
Germany

JANET SHELLENBERGER, RN, PhD
Health Education Consultant, Ministry of Education
Lao PDR
Laos

DIANE SZWEZ, RN, BS
Student, School of Nursing, University of Connecticut
Storrs, Connecticut
Russia, Ukraine

LESLEY WILLCOXSON, PhD
Coordinator, Monash-ANZ Centre for International Briefing
Melbourne, Victoria, Australia
Australia

◆ SPECIAL RECOGNITION

Several sources were especially helpful in the preparation of this manuscript and deserve special recognition for their contributions.

Byrne DMT, editor-in-chief: *NBC News, Rand McNally world atlas & almanac,* 1992. This source is cited for demographic and geographic data.

Dardick KR, Neumann HH: *Foreign travel & immunization guide,* ed 13, Oradell, NJ, 1990, Medical Economics Books. This source is cited for endemic diseases.

Galazka A: Medical Officer, Expanded Programme on Immunization, World Health Organization, Geneva, 1991. This source is cited for the most recent immunization schedules provided to the World Health Organization by the country.

Hoffman MS, editor: *The world almanac,* New York, 1989, Pharos Books. This source is cited for demographic and geographic data.

Johnson O, editor: *The 1992 information please almanac,* Boston, 1992, Houghton Mifflin. This source is cited for demographic and geographic data.

PC Globe, Tempe, 1989, PC Globe. This source is cited for information on common languages, ethnic groups, and religions.

As we approach the twenty-first century, health care professionals in all areas of practice are perched on the cutting edge of enormous demographic, social, and cultural change. Many of these changes will play a dramatic role in the clients' health care beliefs and practices and in their health care needs.

It has often been said that "demography is destiny." Evidence of demographic change in the United States can be verified in two ways: by comparing the census of 1990 with that of 1980 and by examining immigration profiles. Comparing information in the 1990 census with that in the 1980 census will reveal how the people of our nation are changing. For example, the European majority has shrunk by at least 3%. When discussing immigration (legal and illegal), it must be remembered that most people in this country are immigrants, or their ancestors were immigrants. The early waves of immigrants were predominantly European. People are now pouring into this country from all the nations of the world, with the largest numbers coming from Asia and from the Americas, especially Mexico and Central America.

The clients that health care practitioners care for are frequently people who are newcomers and who are neither acculturated nor assimilated into the cultural values of the dominant culture. Language, too, is an issue because the probability that the new immigrants do not speak English is high. Furthermore, every immigrant group has brought with them their own culture, beliefs, and attitudes in respect to health and illness.

The role that culture plays in health care practices can be described in numerous ways. Imagine, for a moment, a kaleidoscope. When the kaleidoscope is turned, countless, colorful pieces of glass at one end reflect in mirrors to create an infinite number of designs. The single piece of glass remains the same; that is, the surface maintains its color, shape, and size; yet, as it turns around, it seems to change within the context of the larger whole. This *whole* constantly changes as it turns and is reflected in the mirrors to form the designs; so it is, too, with a given person or family. The person may have his or her own health and illness beliefs and practices that are reflective of the larger group's original cultural identity. These beliefs and practices may be in constant change; however, they still have similarities within the group context.

Indeed, countless health beliefs and practices are manifested by people from different backgrounds that *may* be observed among people who are members of the various ethnic/cultural communities of the United States. The word *may* must be used to prevent any kind of stereotyping, for the range of health definitions, beliefs, and practices is infinite. Individual differences exist both within a given group of people and among groups. However, some discernible commonalities also exist in the connotations of health and illness and in health-related practices. People who have maintained traditional belief systems often have culturally based or folk beliefs that determine the definitions of health and illness and subsequent practices. These beliefs may include the client's use of protective objects, substances, or religious practices to prevent and treat illness.

Other cultural factors include:
- Communication—both verbal and nonverbal
- Space—the distances that people must maintain while interacting with one another
- Time orientation—whether people from the given cultural group are present, past, or future oriented

The clients who enter this country from nations such as Brunei, Guinea-Bissau, or Kuwait may cause the practitioner concern about how to meet their health care needs. The practitioner may ask: Who is this person? Where is his or her country of origin located? What is his or her ethnic/cultural heritage? What are some of the religious beliefs that may affect care?

The *Pocket Guide to Cultural Assessment* can serve health care professionals well. It provides an introduction to people who originate in over 150 of the earth's nations, from **A,** Afghanistan, to **Z,** Zimbabwe. It provides such information as the geographic location of the country, the major spoken languages, the health and illness practices of the dominant groups of people, the diverse ethnic groups, and various rites, such as birth and death. The guide can be used most productively in an introductory manner and is a point of entry to discover who the client may be and where he or she may have originated.

Health care professionals who practice in all clinical areas and roles must continually nourish awareness of and sensitivity for the cultural needs of clients and families. Awareness of changing demographic and immigration trends, a sensitivity for cultural-based health traditions, an ability to communicate in another language (either by speaking a second language or by using competent interpreters), and an awareness of the clients' beliefs vis-à-vis space and time orientation are several of the ongoing activities that will enhance the transcultural practice of nursing and medical care. *The frequent use of this* Pocket Guide to Cultural Assessment *is step one.*

Rachel E. Spector, PhD, RN, CTN

Associate Professor
Boston College School of Nursing
Chestnut Hill, Massachusetts

I agree with the present trend in transcultural theory, which posits that individuals within any given culture vary markedly. The earth is populated with a vast mosaic of cultures representing every imaginable variety of learned and environmentally generated beliefs and practices. Culture is deeply ingrained and comfortable for most, guiding conscious activities, covert activities, and behaviors in their daily lives during times of health or times of illness. Culture is also a dynamic influence that meets the changing needs of groups.

One of the weaknesses of a guide such as this is that the reader may have a tendency to drift into assumptions that involve *stereotyping*. The reader is *strongly cautioned against* assuming that people from one country or geographic area are clones of one another and that they hold the same beliefs as those held by their neighbors. The borders of countries are politically determined and do not represent boundaries for cultural values. The different values found within one culture may be as numerous as the variations found when comparing two different cultures. Stewart and Bennett[1] remind us that the tendency to stereotype can be overcome

by approaching every cross-cultural situation as a kind of experiment. They should assume that some kind of cultural difference exists but that the nature of the difference is unclear. Using available generalizations about the other culture, they can formulate a hypothesis and then test it for accuracy. . . . The hypothesis should be tested by acting tentatively as if it were accurate and by watching carefully to see what happens. . . . Stewart EC, Bennett MJ.

Galanti[2] makes an effective distinction between stereotyping and generalizing in the story of Rosa, a Mexican woman: "(If) I say to myself, Rosa is Mexican, she must have a large family, I am stereotyping her." Stereotyping closes my mind to potential differences: "But if I think Mexicans often have large families, I wonder if Rosa does, I am asking a generalization," and I remain receptive to further questioning and assessment of Rosa as a unique individual.

I proceeded with this project because of the reality of the workaday world. A care provider cannot say to a patient from an unfamiliar culture, "Excuse me. I'll be back in a few hours (or a few days) after I learn about your culture." Information is scattered throughout a multitude of journals and books, and most of those are not readily accessible. (Note: "No data available" indicates that inquiries were made with World Health Organization, Cumulative Index to Nursing and Allied Health Literature, or National Library of Medicine, and no information was available.)

This guide places some basic information about people in the countries of our world at your fingertips—*where you need it.* I researched the National Library of Medicine database and the Cumulative Index of Nursing and Allied Health Literature (CINAHL). People from various countries and health care professionals who have worked extensively abroad were interviewed and are listed as contributors. The Intercultural Communication Institute library in Portland, Oregon, provided data not yet uncovered by health professionals. Because this search was limited to material written in English, and because interviews did not always furnish complete data, some categories are missing for many countries. The information categories that are incorporated in this guide often describe the impact that culture has on health care delivery and were gleaned from my transcultural practice and teaching.

Only information about the dominant culture of a country is presented. Deciding which culture dominates in a particular country was a difficult task. Most countries include numerous ethnic or racial groups, and including all of them would have resulted in a multivolume encyclopedia that would have been beyond the scope of this guide. The United States and Canada require more comprehensive data for the North American health care professional and therefore are not included in this publication. As this guide was being researched and written, enormous changes were occurring in several countries: the former Soviet Union, Yugoslavia, and

Czechoslovakia. The most current information available at the time of writing is included. The reader is referred to the news media to ascertain the latest political boundaries.

The purpose of this guide is to help focus the reader's attention on the potential variations a culturally diverse client may *or may not* exhibit. It is based on generalizations, and the user should not interpret the material to draw stereotypic conclusions. Consult this guide when you are faced with someone from an unfamiliar culture. Use this guide to increase your awareness and understanding quickly and efficiently of *potential* similarities and differences in a particular culture: the generalizations. Without an understanding of cultural patterns in a patient's behavior the caregiver will not know how to assess the patient effectively. It is a *must* to be culturally competent with patients that you routinely encounter in your practice. Cultural competence with many cultures is an unrealistic expectation. Also, not to use a guide such as this for fear of stereotyping impedes movement toward delivery of culturally relevant health care. I am willing to risk criticism for stereotyping; in return, I ask the user to build thoughtfully on the information inside these pages with an individualized cultural assessment.

The following good assessment guides are available:

Leininger MM: Leininger's acculturation health care assessment tool for cultural patterns in traditional and nontraditional lifeways, *J Transcultural Nurs* 2(2):40, 1991.

Orque MS, Block B, Monrroy KSA: *Block's ethnic-cultural assessment guide: ethnic nursing care: a multicultural approach,* St Louis, 1983, Mosby.

Tripp-Reimer T: *Cultural assessment.* In Bellack JP, Bamford PA: *Nursing assessment: a multidimensional approach,* Monterey, Calif, 1984, Wadsworth.

REFERENCES

1. Stewart EC, Bennett MJ: *American cultural patterns: a cross-cultural perspective,* Yarmouth, Me, 1991, Intercultural Press, pp 167-168.
2. Galanti GA: *Caring for patients from different cultures,* Philadelphia, 1991, University of Pennsylvania Press, p 2.

Elaine M. Geissler

COUNTRIES

◆ AFGHANISTAN

MAP PAGE (264)

Location: Afghanistan is split east to west by the Hindu Kush mountain range, wedged between the former Soviet Union, China, Pakistan, and Iran. With the exception of the southwest, most of the country is covered by high, snowcapped mountains and deep valleys.

Major Languages	Ethnic Groups		Major Religions	
Pushtu	Pashtun	50%	Sunni Muslim	74%
Dari Persian	Tajik	25%	Shi'a Muslim	15%
Turkish	Uzbek	9%	Other	11%
Baluchi	Hazara	9%		
Pashai	Other	7%		

Predominant Sick Care Practices: Magico-religious. Charms and amulets are worn to ward off evil spirits. People of this region believe that evil spirits manifest in a number of central nervous system diseases.

Ethnic/Race Specific or Endemic Diseases: ENDEMIC: Chloroquine-resistant malaria is limited to a belt in the east and rare in Kabul; gastroenteritis among infants during the summer; and cutaneous leishmaniasis. RISK: Intestinal obstruction caused by ascariasis.

Dominance Patterns: Females are subservient to males. Polygamy is practiced. Most women wear the traditional veil.

Birth Rites: Infant and maternal mortality rates are high. Tetanus neonatorum is one cause of infant death. Most births are assisted by traditional birth attendants (dais); many dais are given some basic training.

Death Rites: Relatives and friends come to the home of the family to express sympathy and, if money is needed, contribute. The body remains in the home with a mullah (priest) or close relatives, who read from the Koran throughout the night. The body is washed by relatives or specialists, wrapped in new white clothing, and placed in a coffin. The body must be buried (not cremated) within 24 hours. Two days after the funeral, a ceremony is held in the mosque or house of the deceased and is followed by a meal.

Food Practices and Intolerances: Because food is not inspected for contaminates, boiled water and milk products are advised. Using the hands to eat is acceptable.

Infant Feeding Practices: Breastfeeding is almost universal and continues, sometimes supplemented with bottle feeding (introduced at 6 months), until the next pregnancy. Tea and "zoof" (fried Linn seeds and cooking oil) provide energy and fat-soluble vitamins. These are given to the majority of infants. Contaminated pacifier nipples contribute to the occurrence of diarrhea and malnutrition. Two thirds of the children show signs of protein-energy malnutrition; one fifth show severe malnutrition.

Child Rearing Practices: Children are an economic asset; they work to supplement the household income. Child labor is more common in rural areas and among male children.

National Childhood Immunizations: OPV-1 at 3 months; OPV-2 at 6 months; and OPV-3 at 9 months. The inadequacy of Afghanistan's immunization program is in the morbidity and mortality figures.

BIBLIOGRAPHY

Li GR: *Funeral practices,* New York, World Relief, n.d.

Singh M: Health status of children in Afghanistan, *J Indian Acad Pediatr* 20(5):317, 1983.

Storti C: *The art of crossing cultures,* Yarmouth, Me, 1990, Intercultural Press.

◆ ALBANIA

MAP PAGE (258)

Location: Situated on the eastern shore of the Adriatic Sea with Greece to the south, Albania is a mountainous (3000 feet; 914 m) country with a marshy coastal plain.

Major Language	Ethnic Groups		Major Religions	
Albanian	Albanian	96%	Muslim	70%
	Greek and		Albanian	
	Other	4%	Orthodox	20%
			Catholic	10%

Death Rites: Muslims believe that the human body belongs to God, and organ donations or transplants are forbidden. Muslim physicians may recommend transfusions to save lives. Autopsy is uncommon because the deceased must be buried intact. Cremation is not permitted. For Muslim burial the body is wrapped in special pieces of cloth and buried without a coffin in the ground.

National Childhood Immunizations: DPT-1 at 2 months; DPT-2 at 4 months; DPT-3 at 6 months; DPT boosters at 2 and 6 years; DT at 15 years; OPV-1 at 2 months; OPV-2 at 4 months; OPV-3 at 6 months; OPV boosters at 18 months and 6 years; measles between 9 and 12 months; rubella and mumps at 12 months; BCG between 13 and 15 months, 6 and 7 years, 11 and 12 years, and 17 and 18 years.

BIBLIOGRAPHY

Ross HM: Societal/cultural views regarding death and dying, *Top Clin Nurs* 1(1):1, 1981.
USA Today: June 12, 1991.

◆ ALGERIA

MAP PAGE (260)

Location: Located in North Africa, Algeria is bordered on the west by Morocco and on the east by Tunisia and Libya. Small areas near the Mediterranean coast are low plains. The country is 68% plateau (between 2625 and 5250 feet; 800 and 1600 m).

Major Languages	Ethnic Groups		Major Religions	
Arabic	Arab Berber	99%	Sunni	
French	European		Muslim	99%
Berber	and		Other	1%
	Other	1%		

Ethnic/Race Specific or Endemic Diseases: RISK: Schistosomiasis and chloroquine-sensitive malaria; no risk in urban areas; limited risk in the Sahara.

Families' Role in Hospital Care: Family members or close friends often accompany the patient and expect to participate in care, taking a vigilant supervisory role.

Dominance Patterns: Males dominate; sex roles are clearly and rigidly defined. Women's faces usually are veiled.

Pain Reactions: Those who accept the technology of western medicine expect and request immediate pain relief. Energy is conserved for recovery, contraindicating therapies involving exertion. Pain is expressed only in private or with close relatives or friends; pain during labor and delivery is expressive.

Birth Rites: Fathers are not present during delivery. Babies are wrapped tightly in swaddling clothes to protect them physically and psychologically.

Death Rites: Muslim belief forbids organ donation or transplants. Muslim physicians may recommend transfusions to save lives. Autopsy is uncommon because the deceased must be buried intact. Cremation is not permitted. For Muslim burial the body is wrapped in special pieces of cloth and buried without a coffin in the ground.

Food Practices and Intolerances: Lamb and chicken are eaten frequently. Pork, carrion, and blood are forbidden. Food usually is spicy. Ramadan fasting is practiced with exemptions for the sick and for children.

Infant Feeding Practices: Breastfeeding is common. Mothers may wean the infant abruptly.

National Childhood Immunizations: BCG; DPT-1; DPT-2; DPT-3; DPT booster; measles at 9 months; OPV at birth: OPV-1; OPV-2; OPV-3; OPV booster.

Other Characteristics: Hope, optimism, and the positive advantages of treatment should be stressed when discussing outcomes.

BIBLIOGRAPHY

Green J: Death with dignity—Islam, *Nurs Times* 85(5):56, 1989.

Reizian A, Meleis AI: Arab-Americans' perceptions of and responses to pain, *Crit Care Nurse* 6(6):30, 1986.

Ross HM: Societal/cultural views regarding death and dying, *Top Clin Nurs* 1(1):1, 1981.

Taylor VL, editor: *Culturgrams: the nations around us,* Provo, Utah, 1987, Brigham Young University, David M. Kennedy Center for International Studies.

Zémor O: Midwives in Algeria, *World Health* Dec:15, 1988.

◆ ANDORRA

MAP PAGE (258)

Location: Andorra is a coprincipality situated high in the Pyrenees Mountains on the French/Spanish border.

Major Languages	Ethnic Groups		Major Religions	
Catalan	Spanish	61%	Catholic	99%
French	Andorran	30%	Other	1%
Castilian Spanish	French	6%		
	Other	3%		

BIBLIOGRAPHY
No data located.

◆ ANGOLA

MAP PAGE (261)

Location: Angola extends for more than 1000 miles (1609 km) along the South Atlantic in southwestern Africa. A plateau, averaging 6000 feet (1829 m) in height, rises abruptly from the coastal lowlands. Most of the land is desert or savanna.

Major Languages	Ethnic Groups		Major Religions	
Portuguese	Ovimbundu	38%	Catholic	68%
Bantu Languages	Kimbundu	23%	Protestant	20%
	Bakongo	13%	Other	12%
	Mestizo	2%		
	European and Other	24%		

Ethnic/Race Specific or Endemic Diseases: ACTIVE: Cholera and yellow fever. **ENDEMIC:** Chloroquine-resistant malaria. **RISK:** Schistosomiasis.

Birth Rites: Nurses and midwives perform most maternity care.

National Childhood Immunizations: BCG at birth; DPT-1 at 2 months; DPT-2 at 3 months; DPT-3 at 4 months; DPT booster; measles at 9 months; OPV at birth; OPV-1 at 2 months; OPV-2 at 3 months; OPV-3 at 4 months; OPV booster.

BIBLIOGRAPHY

Raisler J: Anatomy of a training seminar: teaching and learning in Angola, *J Nurse Midwife* 34(1):36, 1989.

◆ **ANTIGUA AND BARBUDA**

MAP PAGE (257)

Location: Antigua, the larger of these two eastern Caribbean islands, is low-lying, deforested, and subject to droughts. Barbuda is a wooded, coral island.

Major Languages	Ethnic Groups		Major Religions	
English	African	96%	Anglican	98%
Local Languages	Other	4%	Other	2%

Other Characteristics: Several people may engage in simultaneous conversations, with frequent interruptions, loud verbal battles, repetition, cursing, and boasting. Such discourse is valued as a normal part of interpersonal relationships.

BIBLIOGRAPHY

Menyuk P, Menyuk D: *Communicative competence: a historical and cultural perspective.* In Wurzel JS: *Toward multiculturalism,* Yarmouth, Me, 1988, Intercultural Press.

◆ ARGENTINA

MAP PAGE (258)

Location: Argentina, a land of plains from the Atlantic to the Chilean border, also has the high peaks of the Andes. The north is swampy, the central populated area has fertile land for agriculture or grazing. The south boasts Patagonia, with its cool, arid steppes. Many Argentineans are of Italian descent. Life expectancy is one of the highest in South America; the standard of living is generally high.

Major Languages	Ethnic Groups		Major Religions	
Spanish	White	85%	Catholic	90%
English	Native		Protestant	2%
Italian	American		Jewish	2%
German	and Mestizo	15%	Other	6%
French				

Ethnic/Race Specific or Endemic Diseases: ENDEMIC: Chloroquine-sensitive malaria is present; however, it is not found in urban areas. RISK: Argentine hemorrhagic fever in four provinces.

Dominance Patterns: Deference is given to the father; however, he considers the opinions of the rest of the family.

Eye Contact Practices: Eye contact is maintained.

Touch Practices: Males may touch while in conversation.

Perceptions of Time: A relaxed attitude toward punctuality exists.

Food Practices and Intolerances: The staple food for many is beef; it is eaten three times a day.

National Childhood Immunizations: DPT-1 at 2 months; DPT-2 at 4 months; DPT-3 at 6 months; DPT boosters at 18 months and 6 years; OPV-1 at 2 months; OPV-2 at 4 months; OPV-3 at 6 months; OPV boosters at 18 months and 6 years; measles at 12 months; BCG at birth; if warranted, BCG at 6 years and 16 years.

BIBLIOGRAPHY

Latin America: intercultural experiential learning aid, Provo, Utah, 1976, Language Research Center, Brigham Young University.

Taylor VL, editor: *Culturgrams: the nations around us,* Provo, Utah, 1987, Brigham Young University, David M. Kennedy Center for International Studies.

U.S. Agency of International Development: Agency program fights Argentine virus, *Front Lines* 31(10):4, 1991.

◆ AUSTRALIA

MAP PAGE (255)

Location: Australia is the only country that occupies a complete continent. Its western half is a desert plateau that includes the Great Victoria Desert to the south and the Great Sandy Desert to the north. The Great Barrier Reef, 1245 miles (2000 km) long, lies along the northeast coast. Aborigines were the only inhabitants when the Dutch discovered parts of the continent in 1623.

Major Languages	Ethnic Groups		Major Religions	
English	White	95%	Anglican	26%
Aborigine	Asian	4%	Catholic	26%
	Aborigine		Other	
	and Other	1%	Christian	24%
			Other	24%

With large numbers of aboriginals and immigrants, many Australians come from a non-English-speaking background.

Predominant Sick Care Practices: Biomedical.

Health Care Beliefs: Active involvement; health promotion is important.

Health Team Relationships: National socialized medicine is in force, with health care available to all; it is funded by a 2% levy on salaries. Respect for authority figures (physicians, in particular) is not strong. Patients may question diagnoses. Physicians encourage patients to express their feelings.

Families' Role in Hospital Care: To maintain the family atmosphere, families are encouraged to feed, bathe, and care for their children in some hospitals.

Dominance Patterns: The male has a strong role, especially in making decisions for the family. The female is the primary child care giver, even though she may be working. The term "mate" is used to indicate comaraderie among males.

Eye Contact Practices: A combination of direct eye contact and looking away shows interest; however, direct eye contact may not be sustained.

Touch Practices: Demonstrations of familiarity (e.g., hugging) are avoided, especially among males. Today females touch frequently when greeting or at departure.

Perceptions of Time: Being punctual for appointments is important; being punctual for social functions is viewed more leniently. Orientation lies in the present, with less worrying about the future. Long-term health promotion activities, such as smoking cessation or reducing high cholesterol levels, are not associated with future benefits.

Pain Reactions: Pain is expressed verbally and within limits.

Birth Rites: A physician usually delivers, but home birth, alternative birthing centers, and use of midwives are increasing. Lamaze method and Alexander technique are common. The father is usually present at the birth.

Death Rites: Cremation and burial are both practiced. The family usually does not see the body, and no wake is held. Grieving is reserved: crying with no wailing. Health care practitioners are expected to help families through the stages of grief, to provide privacy, to be sensitive to the family's desires regarding arrangements for an autopsy, for the mortuary, for viewing the body (if desired), and for the funeral.

Food Practices and Intolerances: Large amounts of beef and dairy products are consumed, with a current tendency toward ingesting less in dairy fats and more in polyunsaturated fats. The consumption of beer is one of the highest per capita.

Infant Feeding Practices: Breastfeeding is encouraged until the child is between 3 and 6 months.

Child Rearing Practices: Emphasis is placed on discipline. Children are encouraged to develop independence within clearly defined limits and controls.

National Childhood Immunizations: Triple antigen; Sabin; 2 DT boosters; polio; diphtheria; tetanus (encouraged but not required); measles vaccine provided in schools.

Other Characteristics: Large teeth are present, with as many as four extra molars. Incidence of skin cancer is one of the highest in the world. Open expression (bordering on the confrontational) or critical questioning during interactions is commonplace. Disagreement is often a valued basis for conversations, eliciting real interest and respect in the participants. Positioning the thumbs upward is a rude gesture; curling the index finger inward is used only to call animals.

BIBLIOGRAPHY

Ashby MA et al: An inquiry into death and dying at the Adelaide Children's Hospital: a useful model? *Med J Aust* 154(3):165, 1991.
Davis AJ, Slater PV: U.S. and Australian nurses' attitudes and beliefs about the good death, *Image* 21(1):34, 1989.

People to have a voice in health care, Health Victoria Supplement, 1985.

Kanitsaki O: Transcultural nursing: challenge to change, *Austral J Adv Nurs* 5(3):4, 1988.

McCallum LW et al: The Ankall project: a model for the use of volunteers to provide emotional support in terminal illness, *Med J Aust* 151(1):33, 37, 1989.

McKenna B: *Aboriginal culture in the Kimberly region: a guide for health practitioners,* Perth, Australia, 1987, Health Department of Western Australia.

Overfield T: *Biologic variation in health and illness,* Menlo Park, Calif, 1985, Addison-Wesley.

People To People International Citizen Ambassador Program, *J People Transcultur Nurs Deleg Australia & New Zealand,* Spokane, 1987.

Renwick GW: *Australians and North Americans,* Yarmouth, Me, 1980, Intercultural Press.

Singh B, Raphael B: Postdisaster morbidity of the bereaved: a possible role for preventive psychiatry, *J Nerv Ment Dis* 169(4):203, 1981.

Sleed J: Manners abroad need study, Portland, Ore, Newhouse News Service, n.d.

Storti C: *The art of crossing cultures,* Yarmouth, Me, 1990, Intercultural Press.

Taylor VL, editor: *Culturgrams: the nations around us,* Provo, Utah, 1987, Brigham Young University, David M. Kennedy Center for International Studies.

Westbrook MT, Nordholm LA, McGee JE: Cultural differences in reactions to patient behaviour: a comparison of Swedish and Australian health professionals, *Soc Sci Med* 19(9):939, 1984.

Willcoxson L: Contributor.

◆ AUSTRIA

MAP PAGE (258)

Location: This landlocked nation in central Europe includes much of the mountainous territory of the eastern Alps, with many snowfields, glaciers, and snowcapped peaks.

Major Language	Ethnic Groups		Major Religions	
German	German	99%	Catholic	85%
	Slavic and		Protestant	6%
	Other	1%	Other	9%

Health Care Beliefs: Active involvement.

Ethnic/Race Specific or Endemic Diseases: RISK: Rett's syndrome in girls.

Health Team Relationships: Patients may consider titles more important than names and use the terms "doctor" or "nurse" in reference to a health professional. In the bureaucratic health care system, initiative is not rewarded and nurses are expected to follow orders for everything except basic nursing care. Nurses do not give injections. Patients receive sufficient oral drugs for 24 hours and are responsible for taking them. Psychologists enjoy a strong role as health care administrators and teachers.

Dominance Patterns: Because the society is patriarchal, women are influenced by husbands or fathers in areas such as politics.

Touch Practices: Privacy curtains between hospital beds are rare because of the communal living styles.

Perceptions of Time: The past is valued. Traditional approaches to healing are more readily accepted than new procedures or medications. The people also value punctuality.

Birth Rites: Natural childbirth and the father's presence in the delivery room are becoming more popular.

Food Practices and Intolerances: The main meal is at midday, and a light meal is eaten in early evening, with another at the end of the day.

National Childhood Immunizations: BCG at one week and between 10 and 15 years; DPT-1 at 3 months; DPT-2 at 4 months; DPT-3 at 5 months; DT between 12 and 18 months, at 7 years, and again between 14 and 15 years; TOPV at 4 months, 7 years, and between 14 and 15 years; measles and mumps at 14 months; rubella for girls only at 13 years.

BIBLIOGRAPHY

Boerckel K: Childbirth education in Austria, *Int J Childbirth Educ* 6(1):39, 1991.

Clift JM: Nursing and health services in Austria, *Nurs Admin Q* 16(2):60, 1992.

Galanti GA: *Caring for patients from different cultures,* Philadelphia, 1991, University of Pennsylvania Press.

Language Research Center: *German-speaking people of Europe,* Provo, Utah, 1976, Brigham Young University.

Morris J: Rett's syndrome: a case study, *J Neurosci Nurs* 22(5):285, 1990.

Reeser DS: An international experience: studying health care systems in Austria and Yugoslavia, *Imprint* 32(1):46, 1985.

Taylor VL, editor: *Culturgrams: the nations around us,* Provo, Utah, 1987, Brigham Young University, David M. Kennedy Center for International Studies.

◆ BAHAMAS

MAP PAGE (257)

Location: The Bahamas include about 700 relatively flat islands (22 are inhabited) off the east coast of Florida, with no fresh water streams.

Major Languages	Ethnic Groups		Major Religions	
English	Black	85%	Baptist	29%
Creole	White	15%	Anglican	23%
			Catholic	22%
			Other	26%

Ethnic/Race Specific or Endemic Diseases: AIDS case rate is 66.1/100,000 people.

BIBLIOGRAPHY

Adler MW, editor: Statistics from the World Health Organization and the Centers for Disease Control, *AIDS* 6(10):1229, 1992.

◆ BAHRAIN

MAP PAGE (262)

Location: An archipelago in the Persian Gulf off the coast of Saudi Arabia, the islands are level expanses of sand and rock.

Major Languages	Ethnic Groups		Major Religions	
Arabic	Bahraini	63%	Shi'a Muslim	70%
English	Asian	13%	Sunni Muslim	30%
Farsi	Other			
Urdu	Arab	10%		
	Iranian	8%		
	Other	6%		

Families' Role in Hospital Care: Family members or close friends participate in the patient's care or take a vigilant and supervisory role.

Pain Reactions: Patients expect immediate pain relief and may request it persistently. Therapies requiring exertion are in conflict with the belief in energy conservation for recovery. Pain is expressed privately or only in the company of close relatives and friends. During labor and delivery, pain is expressed.

Death Rites: Muslim belief forbids organ donations and transplants. Muslim physicians may recommend transfusions to save lives. Autopsy is uncommon because the deceased must be buried intact. Cremation is not permitted. For Muslim burial the body is wrapped in special pieces of cloth and buried without a coffin in the ground.

Food Practices and Intolerances: Pork, carrion, and blood are forbidden. Food tends to be spicy. Ramadan fasting is carried out between sunrise and sunset. The sick and children are exempt.

National Childhood Immunizations: OPV-1 at 2 months; OPV-2 at 3 months; OPV-3 at 4 months.

Other Characteristics: Hope, optimism, and the positive advantages of treatment should be stressed when discussing outcomes.

BIBLIOGRAPHY

al Gasseer NH: Experience of menstrual symptoms among Bahraini women, doctoral dissertation, Chicago, 1990, University of Illinois at Chicago.

Green J: Death with dignity—Islam, *Nurs Times* 85(5):56, 1989.

Reizian A, Meleis AI: Arab-Americans' perceptions of and responses to pain, *Crit Care Nurse* 6(6):30, 1986.

Ross HM: Societal/cultural views regarding death and dying, *Top Clin Nurs* 1(1):1, 1981.

◆ BANGLADESH

MAP PAGE (264)

Location: Formerly East Pakistan, Bangladesh is on the northern coast of the Bay of Bengal and is primarily surrounded by India. The country is low-lying (less than 600 feet [183 m]) and subject to tropical monsoons, frequent floods, and famine. It is one of the most heavily populated and poorest countries in the world.

Major Languages	Ethnic Groups		Major Religions	
Bangla (Bengali)	Bengali	98%	Muslim	83%
English	Biharis		Hindu	16%
	and Other	2%	Other	1%

Predominant Sick Care Practices: Biomedical; magico-religious. Evil spirits and God's will are suspected causes of illness. Injections are perceived as a cure for illness. Faith healers, called Fakirs, are used to exorcise the evil air. Fakirs may be preferred because they spend time with patients and do not always charge a fee. They encourage modern treatment as needed.

Health Care Beliefs: Acute sick care.

Ethnic/Race Specific or Endemic Diseases: ENDEMIC: Chloroquine-resistant malaria. RISK: Japanese encephalitis; iodine deficiency disease is severe, resulting in goiter and mental and physical retardation. Dehydration from diarrhea, acute respiratory tract infections, and low birth weight cause many deaths in those under age 5.

Dominance Patterns: In a patriarchal society women's activities may be severely restricted, including physical seclusion.

Birth Rites: Contraceptive practices have increased in recent years. Rural traditional custom requires the mother to reach a water source unaided and to wash herself and her clothing immediately after delivery. The umbilical cord may be cut with the clean inner strip of a bamboo stalk. After delivery, rituals are performed. The mother chants prayers and stays indoors for 7 days. Only the husband may visit. Plum branches are placed on the door of the home to protect against evil spirits, and the Muslim holy man chants the birth announcement.

Death Rites: Muslim belief forbids organ donations or transplants. Muslim physicians may recommend transfusions to save lives. A Holy Iman does not have to be present at death; however, a Muslim may recite the Declaration of the Faith: "There is no God but God and Muhammed is his Messenger." Family members wash the body according to Islamic tradition. Autopsy is uncommon because the deceased must be buried intact. Cremation is not permitted. For Muslim burial the body is wrapped in special pieces of cloth and buried without a coffin in the ground.

Food Practices and Intolerances: Rice gruel is commonly used during illness. Deficiency of iodine in the water and lack of iodized salt cause many children to show signs of iodine deficiency. People in Bangladesh are among the most malnourished in the world.

Infant Feeding Practices: Economically deprived families breastfeed male and female infants the same until supplementary foods are introduced; then male children may receive higher quality supplementary nutrition.

Child Rearing Practices: Economic and cultural influences prompt the allocation of sparse family nutritional and health care resources to boys, resulting in an increased mortality rate in 1- to 4-year-old female children.

National Childhood Immunizations: BCG at birth; DPT at 6 weeks, 10 weeks, and 14 weeks; TT at 15 years; OPV at birth, 4 weeks, and 8 weeks; measles at 9 months.

BIBLIOGRAPHY

Ahmed S: A birth in Bangladesh, *Midwives Chron and Nurs Notes* 101(1203):98, 1988.

Chowdhury AM et al: Oral rehydration therapy: a community trial comparing the acceptability of homemade sucrose and cereal-based solutions, *Bull World Health Org* 69(2):229, 1991.

Discovery Channel: State of the natural world: children of the monsoon, May 29, 1992.

Koenig MA, D'Souza S: Sex differences in childhood mortality in rural Bangladesh, *Soc Sci Med* 22(1):15, 1986.

Lally MM: Last rites and funeral customs of minority groups, *Midwife Health Visit Comm Nurse* 14(7):224, 1978.

Long N: Mission of the month: Bangladesh, *Front Lines* 32(1):8, 1992.

Nafisa M: Exorcising the evil air, *Nurs Times* 84(27):50, 1988.

Ross HM: Societal/cultural views regarding death and dying, *Top in Clin Nurs* 1(1):1, 1981.

◆ BARBADOS

MAP PAGE (257)

Location: An Atlantic island, Barbados lies 300 miles (483 km) north of Venezuela. The island is 21 miles (34 km) long and 14 miles (23 km) at its widest point. The country is one of the better developed English-speaking Caribbean nations, with a high population density and demographic characteristics consistent with developed countries.

Major Language	Ethnic Groups		Major Religions	
English	African	80%	Anglican	70%
	Mixed	16%	Methodist	9%
	European	4%	Catholic	4%
			Other	17%

Health Care Beliefs: Active involvement.

Ethnic/Race Specific or Endemic Diseases: AIDS case rate is 23.9/100,000 people.

Dominance Patterns: The assumption that strong extended family support systems exist here may not be true. The elderly are cared for in institutions or small one- or two-person households.

Child Rearing Practices: The majority of adults generally approve of corporal punishment, unless it is excessive or self-serving.

BIBLIOGRAPHY

Adler MW, editor: Statistics from the World Health Organization and the Centers for Disease Control, *AIDS* 6(10):1229, 1992.

Brathwaite FS: The elderly in Barbados: problems and policies, *Bull Pan Amer Health Org* 24(3):314, 1990.

Lyte V: Island of innovation: nurse training in Barbados, *Nurs Times* 86(49):44, 1990.

Payne MA: Use and abuse of corporal punishment: a Caribbean view, *Child Abuse Negl* 13(3):1389, 1989.

◆ BELGIUM

MAP PAGE (258)

Location: Belgium, a neighbor of France, West Germany, the Netherlands, and Luxembourg, has an opening onto the North Sea. The land is generally flat with a system of dikes and sea walls along the coast that prevent tidal flooding. Regionalism based on language (Flemish [Dutch] in the north and French in the south) remains the most powerful issue in contemporary Belgium.

Major Languages	Ethnic Groups		Major Religions	
Flemish	Fleming	55%	Catholic	75%
French	Walloon	33%	Protestant	25%
German	Other	12%		

Touch Practices: A handshake or three kisses on the cheek for greeting and leave-taking is common.

Perceptions of Time: Punctuality is practiced.

Food Practices and Intolerances: The main meal is the evening meal. Staples include cheese, bread, fruit, and vegetables, with wine a common beverage.

Other Characteristics: Carrying on a conversation while hands are in the pockets or pointing with a finger is not acceptable.

BIBLIOGRAPHY

Axtell RE, editor: *Do's and taboos around the world,* ed 2, New York, 1990, A Benjamin Book, John Wiley & Sons.

Glen S: A family affair: the health of children and their families: paediatric nurses in Denmark, France, Belgium, and Holland, *Nurs Mirror* 155(24):24, 1982.

Smoyak S: Psychosocial nursing in Belgium, *J Psychosoc Nurs Ment Health Serv* 22(5):35, 1984.

Tyler L, editor: *Culturgrams: the nations around us,* Provo, Utah, 1987, David M. Kennedy Center for International Studies, Brigham Young University.

Wilson H: Community nursing in Belgium, *Nurs Times* 86(29):56, 1990.

◆ BELIZE

MAP PAGE (256)

Location: This Central American nation (formerly British Honduras), faces the Caribbean Sea to the east and is bounded by the Republics of Mexico and Guatemala. The coastline, just a few feet above sea level, is flat, swampy, and fringed by islets (called "cayes") and a barrier reef — the longest in the Western Hemisphere. In the west and south the terrain rises gradually to its highest peak at 3559 feet (1085 m). In this subtropical climate, the rivers are numerous. Although it is surrounded by Spanish-speaking Central American countries, Belize's links to English-speaking eastern Caribbean islands and to Britain remain strong.

Major Languages	Ethnic Groups		Major Religions	
English	Creole	52%	Catholic	62%
Spanish	Mestizo	32%	Protestant	28%
Garifuna	Garifuna	8%	Other	10%
Maya	Other	8%		
Ketchi				
Creole				

Predominant Sick Care Practices: Biomedical; magico-religious. Women of Obeah belief read cards. Dream Books may be consulted to interpret the significance of dreams. The evil eye, mal ojo, is a commonly held belief. Among women the expression "cut your eye at someone" means casting the evil eye. Family herb recipes are often tried before or with biomedical treatment. Nurses and physicians are sought for advice and care.

Health Care Beliefs: Passive role; acute sick care. Regular physical examinations are usually not practiced.

Ethnic/Race Specific or Endemic Diseases: ENDEMIC: Chloroquine-sensitive malaria is found (no risk in urban areas). RISK: Schistosomiasis, keloids, sickle cell anemia, and hypertension are reported.

Health Team Relationships: The physician usually is not questioned by patients. Physician/nurse relationships are superior/subordinate (respectively) relationships. Female chaperons are often present when female patients have physical examinations by male physicians. Male nurses usually do not give intimate physical care to females.

Families' Role in Hospital Care: Families are encouraged to assist with the patient's care and act as advocates. Some families bring food to the patient daily. Chronically ill elderly are often cared for at home; however, they are hospitalized in acute illness. The mentally ill are hospitalized because families are hesitant to care for them at home.

Dominance Patterns: This society is a matriarchal one.

Eye Contact Practices: Many persons do not maintain direct eye contact, especially with authority figures.

Touch Practices: Greetings are usually formal.

Perceptions of Time: The people adhere to schedules.

Pain Reactions: Expressive reactions predominate. Cancer is usually suspected if a reason for the pain cannot be found. It is believed that if pain is denied, it will go away. Before medical aid is sought, home remedies or over-the-counter medications are used. Beliefs include that dark rum relieves headache; hot Coca-Cola or pure lime juice relieves diarrhea; hot food, cold drink, and heavy food are avoided at night to ward off colic and nightmares. Bones of spoiled fish are used to make a soup believed to cure sickness caused by having ingested spoiled fish.

Birth Rites: Half of children are born out-of-wedlock and are called "outside children." Until the early 1960s, newborn babies were christened before relatives or friends were allowed to visit because it was believed that babies not yet christened could be "overlooked" or given the bad eye. In addition to nurse midwives, Belize has a 4-month program for traditional birth attendants (nannies), who are recognized as primary health care workers by the Ministry of Health.

Death Rites: People are demonstrative in their expressions of grief. A spectacular funeral procession includes many cars and people.

Food Practices and Intolerances: Rice, red beans, and fish are food staples that are highly seasoned with pepper. The diet is high in carbohydrates.

Infant Feeding Practices: Although breastfeeding is encouraged, bottle feeding for 3 years is preferred.

Child Rearing Practices: Children are raised with strict discipline until the boys are 13 years and the girls are 16 years. Grandmothers are frequently involved in child care. Disposable diapers are used; however, in rural areas cloth diapers or bare bottoms are the custom. Toilet training begins as soon as the child can sit up. In school, sex education is presented co-educationally to 10- to 12-year-old boys and girls.

National Childhood Immunizations: The belief persists that immunizations make children ill.

Other Characteristics: In 1990 the population estimate was 184,000 people; 44% were 14 years or younger, and 5.6% were 65 years or older. The country has neither a medical school nor a national health insurance. Skin color and/or physical features may influence status and opportunity.

BIBLIOGRAPHY

Belize Information Service and Central Statistics Office: *Belize in figures, 1991,* Belize, 1991, Government Printery.

Buhler RO: Belizean folk remedies, *National Studies* 3(2):17, 1975.

Cody E: Belize: A different beat, The Washington Post, p. A14, Sept 30, 1991.

Dobson N: *History of Belize,* Port of Spain, 1973, Longman Caribbean.

Fact Sheet: Belize, Belize, 1989, Government Information Service.

Herrmann EK: Contributor.

Herrmann EK: *Origins of tomorrow: a history of Belizean nursing education,* Belize, 1985, Ministry of Health.

Holland J: Promoting primary health in Belize, *Health Visit* 56(11):400, 1983.

Johnson JD et al: Communication factors related to closer international ties: an extension of a model in Belize, *Internat J Intercult Relations* 13(1):1, 1989.

Johnson L: Belizean Medical Student at the University of the West Indies. Personal communication to EK Herrmann, 1989.

Johnson S: Principal Nursing Officer, Belize. Personal communications to EK Herrmann, Feb 1990, July 1991.

Robbins W: Health care Belize style: have clinic, will travel, *Front Nurs Serv Q Bull* 63(2):12, 1987.

◆ BENIN

MAP PAGE (260)

Location: Benin (formerly Dahomey), located in West Africa on the Gulf of Guinea, is one of the smallest and most densely populated countries in Africa. A narrow coastal strip of land rises to a swampy, forested plateau, with highlands to the north.

Major Languages	Ethnic Groups		Major Religions	
French	African	99%	Indigenous	
Fon	European	1%	Beliefs	70%
Yoruba			Muslim	15%
Other			Christian	15%

Predominant Sick Care Practices: Magico-religious. The practice of folk healers (medicine people) is often specialized.

Ethnic/Race Specific or Endemic Diseases: ENDEMIC: Yellow fever; chloroquine-resistant malaria.

Birth Rites: Indigenous and government-trained nurse midwives provide care during deliveries; however, some indigenous midwives exclude duties that involve washing the baby or cutting the umbilical cord. During birth, the kneeling position is used; most deliveries take place at home. Female circumcision may be performed; infanticide may occur in rural areas, if an infant displays signs of witchcraft.

National Childhood Immunizations: BCG at birth; DPT-1 at 1½ months; DPT-2 at 2½ months; DPT-3 at 3½ months, with no booster; measles at 9 months; OPV at birth; OPV-1 at 1½ months; OPV-2 at 2½ months; OPV-3 at 3½ months, with no booster.

BIBLIOGRAPHY

Sargent C: The implications of role expectations for birth assistance among Bariba women, *Soc Sci Med* 16:1483, 1982.

◆ BHUTAN

MAP PAGE (264)

Location: Bhutan is a mountainous country on the southeast slope of the Himalayas, bordering Tibet and India. A succession of lofty and rugged mountains reach 24,000 feet (7315 m), separated by deep and sometimes high valleys. A subtropical zone of humid plains exhibits thick tropical forests. Most people live in the intermediate areas between the plains and the high mountains.

Major Languages	Ethnic Groups		Major Religions	
Dzongkha	Bhote	60%	Buddhist	75%
Nepalese	Nepalese	25%	Hindu	25%
Tibetan Dialects	Other	15%		

Predominant Sick Care Practices: Traditional. People believe that sickness comes to those who have engaged in evil actions. Indian Ayurvedic medicine and Tibetan herb medicine are practiced. People have faith in the local healers.

Health Care Beliefs: Passive role; acute sick care. Events are determined by the fates or the deities and cannot be changed.

Ethnic/Race Specific or Endemic Diseases: ENDEMIC: Chloroquine-resistant malaria in rural areas; respiratory diseases, including tuberculosis; iodine deficiency goiter; leprosy; and vitamin A deficiency in certain areas. RISK: Gastrointestinal diseases are found in young children; parasites are common. Hand washing and sanitary waste disposal are not practiced in some areas, contaminating drinking water. Young women self-inflict burns in response to family quarrels.

Food Practices and Intolerances: Rice is a staple.

National Childhood Immunizations: BCG soon after birth; DPT at 6 weeks, 10 weeks, and 14 weeks; measles at 270 days; OPV at 6 weeks, 10 weeks, and 14 weeks. Because good health results from past virtue, immunizations are not perceived as being able to affect future health.

BIBLIOGRAPHY

Bibbings J: VSO nursing in Bhutan, *Nurs: J Clin Pract Educ Manage* 3(47):9, 1989.
Bibbings J: Wound care in a developing country, *Nurs: J Clin Pract Educ Manage* 4(41):29, 1991.
Clinchy RA: Emergency medicine comes to the Himalayas, *Emergency* Oct:42, 1984.

◆ BOLIVIA

MAP PAGE (258)

Location: Bolivia is landlocked in the heart of South America, with high, cold, dry mountains (Altiplanos) in the west, medium elevation valleys in the middle, and low, wet, hot, forested plains in the east.

Major Languages	Ethnic Groups		Major Religions	
Spanish	Quechua	30%	Catholic	95%
Quechua	Aymara	25%	Indigenous	
Aymara	Mixed	30%	and Other	5%
	European	15%		

Ethnic/Race Specific or Endemic Diseases: RISK: Yellow fever; chloroquine-resistant malaria is present, with no risk in urban areas.

Health Team Relationships: Physicians expect nurses to assume a traditional, passive role.

Eye Contact Practices: Avoiding eye contact during conversations is considered insulting. Eyes and facial expressions often are used to communicate.

Touch Practices: Females who are friends may walk arm-in-arm or hold hands.

Perceptions of Time: Punctuality is flexible.

Death Rites: The Aymara's (a cultural group [Indian] living in mountainous areas) life is built around an acceptance of death.

National Childhood Immunizations: DPT-1 at 3 months; DPT-2 at 6 months; DPT-3 at 9 months; OPV-1 at 3 months; OPV-2 at 6 months; OPV-3 at 9 months; measles at 9 months.

Other Characteristics: Bolivians believe that their country's system of social welfare is one of the best in the world because their benefits are clearly spelled out in the constitution; however, they are not unduly concerned if people do not receive the benefits the constitution promises.

BIBLIOGRAPHY

Bastien JW: The making of a community health worker, *World Health Forum* 11(4):368, 1990.

Fryer ML: Health education through interactive radio: a child-to-child project in Bolivia, *Health Educ Q* 18(1):65, 1991.

Ross HM: Societal/cultural views regarding death and dying, *Top Clin Nurs* 1(1):1, 1981.

Savino MM: The professional nursing role in Cochabamba, Bolivia: clinical nurses' and physicians' perceptions about ideal and actual functioning; identified role problems; and leadership recommendations. Doctoral dissertation, Ithaca, NY, 1988, Cornell University.

Stewart EC, Bennett MJ: *American cultural patterns: a cross-cultural perspective,* rev ed, Yarmouth, Me, 1991, Intercultural Press.

Tyler L: *Culturgrams: the nations around us,* vol 1, Provo, Utah, 1987, David M. Kennedy Center for International Studies, Brigham Young University.

◆ BOTSWANA

MAP PAGE (261)

Location: This south central African country is near-desert, with salt lakes in the north and the Khalahari Desert in a basin on the plateau region. The climate is subtropical. Rural people live in large villages. Most people live in the eastern part of the nation where greater rainfall produces better grazing land.

Major Languages	Ethnic Groups		Major Religions	
English	Botswana	95%	Indigenous	
se Tswana	Bushmen	4%	Beliefs	50%
	European	1%	Christian	48%

Predominant Sick Care Practices: Biomedical; traditional. Herbalists and diviners are common folk healers; however, herbs are not used for common illnesses. People seek spiritual healers at African Christian churches. The people believe in the practice of sorcery and take daily precautions to protect themselves against jealousy. Folk healers have special areas of expertise, and treatments from two or more systems are not used simultaneously because they can cancel out each other.

Health Care Beliefs: Acute sick care; health promotion is important. Nurses promote preventive, diagnostic, and curative skills.

Ethnic/Race Specific or Endemic Diseases: ENDEMIC: Chloroquine-resistant malaria; schistosomiasis. RISK: Tuberculosis; diarrhea; measles; protein-calorie malnutrition in children.

Health Team Relationships: Nurses have an important role because of the shortage of physicians.

Birth Rites: Eating eggs is avoided during pregnancy. Massage is an assessment procedure used in the perinatal period. Approximately one third of the births occur at home and are often assisted by female family members or traditional, untrained midwives. Animal fat is used to oil the newborn, and the baby's head is shaved after the umbilical cord falls off.

National Childhood Immunizations: BCG at birth; DPT-1 at 2 months; DPT-2 at 3 months; DPT-3 at 4 months; DPT booster at 18 months; DT at 6 years; measles at 9 months; OPV-1 at 2 months; OPV-2 at 3 months; OPV-3 at 4 months; OPV booster at 18 months.

BIBLIOGRAPHY

Anderson S: Traditional maternity care within a bio-social framework, *Int Nurs Rev* 33(4):102, 1986.

Barbee EL: Tensions in the brokerage role: nurses in Botswana, *West J Nurs Res* 9(2):244, 1987.

Beardslee C et al: Nursing care of children in developing countries: issues in Thailand, Botswana, and Jordan, *Rec Adv Nurs* 16:31, 1987.

Kupe SS: A history of the evolution of nursing education in Botswana, 1922-1980, doctoral dissertation, New York, 1987, Columbia University Teachers College.

Ngcongco VN, Stark R: Family nurse practitioners in Botswana: challenges and implications, *Int Nurs Rev* 37(2):239, 1990.

◆ BRAZIL

MAP PAGE (258)

Location: Covering nearly half of South America, Brazil is the fifth largest and the sixth most populous country in the world. Sixty percent of the country is covered by forests.

The Amazon River (3912 miles; 6296 km) and the world's largest tropical rain forest are in Brazil. It reflects African, Indian, and Dutch cultures in the north and northeast and German and Italian influences in the south. São Paulo has one of the largest Japanese communities in the world. A developed country, Brazil has two distinct classes: rich and poor, as well as a small middle class.

Major Languages	Ethnic Groups		Major Religions	
Portuguese	White	55%	Catholic	89%
Spanish	Mixed	38%	Other	11%
English	Black	6%		
French	Other	1%		
German				

Predominant Sick Care Practices: Biomedical, holistic; magico-religious (extensive in interior Brazil). Pharmacies run by doctors of homeopathy are common.

Health Care Beliefs: Active involvement; passive role. A recently inaugurated Unified Health System (SUS) places emphasis on primary health care. Active involvement is practiced by the small, middle-class element, with a more passive role among the poor.

Ethnic/Race Specific or Endemic Diseases: ACTIVE: Cholera. ENDEMIC: Chloroquine-resistant malaria. RISK: Dengue fever; cholera; yellow fever; schistosomiasis; leprosy; diarrhea; parasites; malnutrition. Many people attribute health problems to a malfunctional liver.

Health Team Relationships: The term "doctor" *(dotor)* is used indiscriminately to express respect and affection. Nurses are addressed by a title followed by their first name.

Families' Role in Hospital Care: The family assumes some responsibility for direct care, such as bringing food. Family members may take turns staying with the patient 24 hours a day.

Dominance Patterns: The extended family includes godparents and godchildren. When speaking in the third person, parents are referred to as *senhor* or *senhora*. When more than one last name is used, the mother's name comes first.

Eye Contact Practices: Direct eye contact dominates.

Touch Practices: Women greet by kissing on both cheeks and men shake hands and embrace; however, greeting a professional is limited to a handshake.

Perceptions of Time: Brazilians are casual about punctuality and are oriented to the present. The future is measured in decades or generations, and definitions of early and late are flexible. Arriving late may indicate a successful social standing. Rewards for current activity are preferred over delayed gratification.

Pain Reactions: Pain is expressed vocally. Persons from the interior tend to somatize problems.

Food Practices and Intolerances: Yams, bread, and *cous-cous* are common for breakfast. Noon is the main meal and consists of rice, beans, mashed potatoes, and meat or fish. A light meal is taken around 8 PM.

Infant Feeding Practices: Breastfeeding is short term; São Paulo women breastfeed for a longer term.

Child Rearing Practices: Children are treated affectionately; kissing a child is preceded by inhaling (smelling). Pacifiers are tied to the diaper or kept on a cord around the infant's neck. Grandmothers play an active role in care giving, especially for working mothers. Students attend public high schools for half a day (morning, afternoon, or evening). Children in the lower socioeconomic bracket often work rather than go to school; homeless children are a major concern in large cities.

National Childhood Immunizations: DPT-1 at 2 months; DPT-2 at 4 months; DPT-3 at 6 months; DPT booster at 18 months; OPV-1 at 2 months; OPV-2 at 4 months; OPV-3 at 6 months; OPV boosters at 18 months and 4 years; measles at 9 months; BCG at birth.

Other Characteristics: The finger sign for OK in the United States is a crude sexual invitation in Brazil. The thumbs up sign indicates fine, OK, or great.

BIBLIOGRAPHY

Angels with wet wings won't fly: maternal sentiment in Brazil and the image of neglect, *Cult Med Psychiatry* 12:141, 1988.

Angerami ELS, Puntel de Almeida MC: Nursing administration trends in Brazil, *Nurs Admin Q* 16(2):47, 1992.

Beasley A: Breastfeeding studies: culture, biomedicine, and methodology, *J Hum Lact* 7(1):7, 1991.

Beckmann CA: Maternal-child health in Brazil, *JOGNN* 16(4):238, 1987.

Coler MS: Contributor.

Coler MS, Hafner LP: An intercultural assessment of the type, intensity, and number of crisis precipitating factors in three cultures: United States, Brazil and Taiwan, *Int J Nurs Study* 28(3):223, 1991.

Coler MS et al: Justification for mental health services at the department of nursing, Universidade Federal da Paraiba-Brasil through the utilization of nursing diagnoses and diagnostic categories, *Classif Nurs Diagn Proc Eighth Conf* 165, 1989.

Coler MS et al: A Brazilian study of two diagnoses in the NANDA human response pattern: moving, a transcultural comparison, *Classif Nurs Diagn Proc Ninth Conf* 255, 1991.

Condon JC, Yousef F: *An introduction to intercultural communication,* New York, 1975, Macmillan.

Galanti GA: *Caring for patients from different cultures,* Philadelphia, 1991, University of Pennsylvania Press.

Gorayeb R: Child rearing patterns in Brazil, *Acta Psychiatr Scand Suppl* 344:147, 1988.

Green HB: Temporal attitudes in four Negro subcultures, *Studium Generale* 23(6):571, 1970.

Hartz J: Children in exile, NBC-TV, March 8, 1992.

Hoy R: Health care in Brazil, *Nurs Lond* 3(47):12, 1989.

Kurian GT, editor: *Encyclopedia of the third world,* ed 4, vol 1, New York, 1992, Facts of Life.

Language Research Center: *Brazil: intercultural experiential learning aid,* Provo, Utah, 1976, Brigham Young University.

Language Research Center: *Latin America: intercultural experiential learning aid,* Provo, Utah, 1976, Brigham Young University.

McGreevey WP: The high costs of health care in Brazil, *Int Nurs Rev* 36(1):13, 1989.

Monteiro CA et al: The recent revival of breast-feeding in the city of São Paulo, Brazil, *Am J Pub Health* 77(8):964, 1987.

Reis HT: Perceptions of time and punctuality in the United States and Brazil, *J Personality Soc Psychol* 38(4):541, 1980.

Schreuders T: Treating leprosy in Amazonas, *Nurs Times* 86(35):60, 1990.

Stewart EC, Bennett MJ: *American cultural patterns: a cross-cultural perspective,* rev ed, Yarmouth, Me, 1991, Intercultural Press.

◆ BRUNEI

MAP PAGE (265)

Location: A thinly populated independent sultanate on the northwest coast of the island of Borneo, Brunei is covered with tropical rain forest.

Major Languages	Ethnic Groups		Major Religions	
Malay	Malay	64%	Muslim	60%
English	Chinese	20%	Buddhist	16%
Brunei-Chinese	Other	16%	Christian	8%
			Other	16%

Death Rites: The Muslim belief forbids organ donations or transplants. Muslim physicians may recommend transfusion to save lives. Autopsy is uncommon because the deceased must be buried intact. Cremation is not permitted. For Muslim burial the body is wrapped in special pieces of cloth and buried without a coffin in the ground.

National Childhood Immunizations: DPT at 3 months, 4½ months, and 6 months, with DT at school entry; polio at 3 months, 4½ months, and 6 months, with boosters at 18 months and 5 years; BCG at birth, 6 years, and 12 years; measles at 9 months; rubella at 12 years for girls.

BIBLIOGRAPHY

Ross HM: Societal/cultural views regarding death and dying, *Top Clin Nurs* 1(1):1, 1981.

◆ BULGARIA

MAP PAGE (258)

Location: Bulgaria is situated on the Black Sea in the eastern part of the Balkan peninsula. Plains cover two thirds of Bulgaria, and one third is mountainous.

Major Language	Ethnic Groups		Major Religions	
Bulgarian	Bulgarian	85%	Bulgarian	
	Turkish	8%	Orthodox	85%
	Gypsy	3%	Muslim	13%
	Macedonian	3%	Other	2%
	Armenian			
	and Other	1%		

Food Practices and Intolerances: Large meals are taken at midday and in the evening. Cheese, yogurt, lamb, and mutton are popular foods.

National Childhood Immunizations: BCG by 2 months and between 6 and 7 years, 10 and 11 years, and at 16 years (for nonreactives); DPT-1 at 3 months; DPT-2 at 4 months; DPT-3 at 5 months; DPT booster at 2 years; DT between 6 and 7 years and at 12 years; OPV-1 at 3 months; OPV-2 at 4 months; OPV-3 at 5 months; OPV boosters at 2 years, 3 years, and between 6 and 7 years; measles and mumps at 13 months; measles again at 25 months.

Other Characteristics: The head motions for yes and no are the opposite of those used in the United States.

BIBLIOGRAPHY

Axtell RE, editor: *Do's and taboos around the world,* ed 2, New York, 1990, John Wiley & Sons.

East meets west: Georgi Georgev talks with Shirley Smoyak: exchanges about the state-of-the-art in mental health, *Psychosoc Nurs Ment Health Serv* 21(11):35, 1983.

Tyler L, editor: *Culturgrams: the nations around us,* Provo, Utah, 1987, The David M. Kennedy Center for International Studies, Brigham Young University.

◆ BURKINA FASO

MAP PAGE (260)

Location: Burkina Faso (formerly Upper Volta) is land-locked in West Africa and consists of plains, low hills, and high savannas, with desert in the north.

Major Languages	Ethnic Groups		Major Religions	
French	Mossi	36%	Indigenous	
Sudanic	Other	64%	Beliefs	65%
Languages			Muslim	25%
			Christian	10%

Ethnic/Race Specific or Endemic Diseases: ENDEMIC: Chloroquine-resistant malaria.

National Childhood Immunizations: BCG at birth; DPT-1 at 2 months; DPT-2 at 3 months; DPT-3 at 4 months; DPT booster at 18 months; yellow fever and measles at 9 months; OPV-1 at 2 months; OPV-2 at 3 months; OPV-3 at 4 months; OPV booster at 18 months.

BIBLIOGRAPHY

Riesman P: On the irrelevance of child rearing practices for the formation of personality: an analysis of childhood, personality, and values in two African communities, *Cult Med Psychiatry* 7(2):103, 1983.

◆ BURMA (MYANMAR)

MAP PAGE (265)

Location: Myanmar occupies the northwest portion of the Indochinese peninsula, with India to the northwest and China to the northeast. It consists of a narrow mountain range, a plateau, and a flat fertile delta.

Major Languages	Ethnic Groups		Major Religions	
Burmese	Burman	68%	Buddhist	85%
Other	Shan	9%	Indigenous	
	Karen	7%	Beliefs	10%
	Raljome	4%	Christian	
	Chinese		and Other	5%
	and Other	12%		

Predominant Sick Care Practices: Biomedical; traditional.

Ethnic/Race Specific or Endemic Diseases: ENDEMIC: Chloroquine-resistant malaria. RISK: Hemoglobin E disease; Japanese encephalitis; leprosy; tuberculosis; goiter; malnutrition; diarrhea; infectious diseases. Intestinal worms frequently are a cause for intestinal surgery in children.

Health Team Relationships: A direct "no" answer to a question is avoided.

Families' Role in Hospital Care: Families stay with the patient in the hospital, performing basic care and providing meals and clean linen. Medicines are purchased by the family and brought to the hospital.

Perceptions of Time: Punctuality is not stressed.

Birth Rites: Family planning is contrary to government policy. Caesarian sections may be performed to avoid the birth of a male child on Saturdays or other inauspicious days. After delivery, the mother remains in the hospital bed for 24 hours; if she delivers at home, she remains in the room where she gave birth for 7 days. She does no work during that time. The mother drinks only boiled water for 45 days after delivery.

Death Rites: Preference is for quality rather than quantity of life because Buddhists believe in reincarnation and less suffering in the next life. The dying are helped to recall past good deeds, enabling them to achieve a fit mental state. Autopsies are permitted; cremation is preferred.

Food Practices and Intolerances: White rice and vegetables are staples.

Infant Feeding Practices: Most infants are breastfed; however, breastfeeding may be delayed because the people believe that colostrum is not good for infants.

National Childhood Immunizations: BCG at 3 months; DPT at 3 months, 5 months, and 7 months; measles at 9 months; OPV at 3 months, 5 months, and 7 months.

BIBLIOGRAPHY

Boyle JS, Andrews MM: *Transcultural concepts in nursing care,* Glenview, Ill, 1989, Scott, Foresman/Little, Brown College Division.

Falla J: Rebels with a cause, *Nurs Times* 84(26):36, 1988.

Forbes C: Burma: the royal and golden country, *Health Visitor* 62(4):119, 1989.

Kington M: Great journeys, PBS-TV, Oct 27, 1991.

Lally MM: Last rites and funeral customs of minority groups, *Midwife Health Visit Com Nurse* 14(7):224, 1978.

Parker T: Born in Burma, *Nurs Times* Jan 14:44, 1987.

Samovar LA, Porter RE: *Intercultural communication: a reader,* Belmont, Calif, 1985, Wadsworth.

◆ BURUNDI

MAP PAGE (261)

Location: Burundi is a high plateau divided by several deep valleys in east central Africa; it is close to the equator. Bantu tribes densely populate the area, ethnic strife and violence exist between the Tutsi and Hutu groups. Burundi is an agricultural nation that experiences famine at times.

Major Languages	Ethnic Groups		Major Religions	
Kirundi	Hutu	85%	Catholic	62%
French	Tutsi	14%	Indigenous	
Swahili	Twa and		Beliefs	32%
	Other	1%	Protestant	5%
			Muslim	1%

Ethnic/Race Specific or Endemic Diseases: ENDEMIC: Yellow fever. RISK: Cholera; chloroquine-resistant malaria.

National Childhood Immunizations: BCG at birth; DPT-1 at 6 weeks; DPT-2 at 10 weeks; DPT-3 at 14 weeks; DPT booster 1 year after DPT-3; measles at 9 months; OPV at birth; OPV-1 at 6 weeks; OPV-2 at 10 weeks; OPV-3 at 14 weeks; OPV booster 1 year after OPV-3.

Other Characteristics: When a person is accused, skillful deception is highly valued.

BIBLIOGRAPHY

Condon JC, Yousef F: *An introduction to intercultural communication,* New York, 1975, Macmillan.

◆ CAMBODIA (KAMPUCHEA)

MAP PAGE (265)

Location: A large alluvial plain on the Indochinese peninsula, Kampuchea is ringed by mountains.

Major Languages	Ethnic Groups		Major Religions	
Khmer	Khmer (Cam-		Theravada	
French	bodian)	90%	Buddhist	95%
	Chinese	5%	Other	5%
	Other	5%		

Predominant Sick Care Practices: Biomedical; holistic; magico-religious; traditional. Biomedical medicine is practiced; however, it does not replace traditional beliefs. Herbal medicine is important to tradition. Most herbal medicines are classified as "cool," while most western medicines are considered "hot." An imbalance in the "hot/cold" theory is believed to be one cause of disease. Traditionally, illness is dealt with through self-care and self-medication. Folk remedies include variations of acupuncture, massage, herbal remedies, and dermabrasive practices such as cupping, pinching, rubbing, and burning.

Health Care Beliefs: Active involvement; acute sick care; health promotion is important. Energizing "hot" forces and calming "cool" forces restore equilibrium in the body and are the treatment goal. The belief in the balance between work and leisure supports laughter as healthy. Unhealthy air currents (bad winds) are thought to get caught inside the body causing illness. Pinching, scratching, or rubbing the area with a coin releases the bad winds. These actions are thought to restore health, leaving marks or red lines on the skin. Accidents are believed to be caused by fate as punishment for past sins; therefore emergency intervention may be considered inappropriate.

Traditionally, mental illness is met with denial. According to beliefs, thinking too much, particularly in periods of stress, creates mental imbalance.

Ethnic/Race Specific or Endemic Diseases: ENDEMIC: Chloroquine-resistant malaria. RISK: Japanese encephalitis; schistosomiasis.

Health Team Relationships: Because physicians are considered experts and authority figures, patients are given little information. Health professionals are respected and patients do not question or oppose them openly; however, patients may not comply with recommended medical regimens. A patient may hide his or her true feelings to avoid disagreement and to appear compliant. This behavior is thought to protect the patient's self-esteem and the health professional's status. Noncompetitive and nonconfrontational approaches by health professionals are indicated. An open show of impatience or anger is culturally inappropriate. Female patients' questions may be answered by the husband. Traditionally, the oldest male in the family makes decisions about health care. A female patient may refuse care from a male health care giver.

Families' Role in Hospital Care: The family is highly valued, and membership within the family is flexible. An understanding of this tradition is helpful to health care professionals.

Dominance Patterns: Decision-making is influenced by the astrologic/lunar calendar. Women defer to men; however, women often control the men, the home, the acute care decisions, and the economic power of the community. The traditional extended family is more important than the individual. The husband is responsible for matters concerning the outside world, and the wife, with all household affairs. Men practice polygamy if the first wife agrees in writing.

Eye Contact Practices: Continuous direct eye contact is disrespectful.

Touch Practices: The head is considered the center of life. It is revered and invasive procedures frighten the patient.

Touching the head is offensive to many. Only parents may be permitted to touch the heads of their children. Touch is a demonstration of love from the family and may be expressed through various means, such as massage or rubbing coins against the skin. Handshaking has gained wide acceptance among men; however, it is not customary among women.

Perceptions of Time: Time is flexible. Planning for the future and keeping appointments are not valued. Taking scheduled medication is not understood because pills are taken only if the patient feels ill.

Pain Reactions: Pain may be severe before relief is requested.

Birth Rites: Because childbirth is thought to be a "cold" condition, warmth is needed to replace lost heat and energy. The mother's head is often covered with blankets or towels. After delivery, the woman may refuse to bathe, drink ice water, or hold her baby and may experience "toa": the period of collapse treated by the restoration of humoral balance and mind/body equilibrium. The woman may have a lying-in period of 1 week to 3 months. The newborn is not given compliments, so that it will not be captured by evil spirits. Buddhist belief in past and future lives places the blame for birth defects on mistakes made in past lives.

Death Rites: The people prefer quality in life rather than quantity because Buddhists believe in reincarnation. They expect less suffering in the next life. Patients prefer to die at home rather than in the hospital. Jewels or portions of rice (depending on the family's financial standing) are placed in the deceased's mouth to help the soul encounter gods or devils and to ensure that the deceased will be wealthy in the next life. Cremation in the temple is preferred, and the deceased's ashes are kept in a pagoda or at home. Immediately following death, monks are called to pray. Neighbors join in the celebrations and may bring small money gifts. The longer and more elaborate a funeral, the more respect is paid to the deceased. White clothes are worn during the 3-month mourning period.

Afterwards, a black armband or black clothing is worn. Some mourners may shave their heads.

Food Practices and Intolerances: Families demonstrate love through food.

Infant Feeding Practices: The female breast is accepted dispassionately as the means of infant feeding; however, colostrum is considered dirty. Breastfeeding may continue up to 3 years, with solids introduced early on.

Child Rearing Practices: The character of an infant's personality is thought to be partially determined by the year and time of day at birth. Methods for calculating the age of an infant may vary as much as 2 years. Babies are frequently fondled, cared for, and carried about by the mother or another woman in the family. Parents are relaxed and enjoy children under 6 years. After that, strict upbringing begins, independence is discouraged, and parents demand obedience. The oldest child, boy or girl, is responsible for younger siblings if the parents die, are old, or are ill. Large families are valued. Between puberty and marriage, the traditional girl spends 1 month in seclusion. She observes many rites, eats a vegetarian diet, remains in her room in the dark, and is visited only by her mother. A child's name may be changed to confuse potential evil spirits.

National Childhood Immunizations: DPT at 3 months, 4 months, and 6 months; DT booster at school entry; polio at 2 months, 3 months, and 6 months; booster at 5 years; BCG at birth and school entry; measles at 8 months.

Other Characteristics: It is believed that a heated coin or one smeared with oil and rubbed vigorously over the body, causing red welts, will draw out illness. The red marks are thought to be evidence that illness is being brought to the surface of the body, proving that those who sustain the marks are indeed ill. Injections also are used and are considered more beneficial to recovery than pills. Wrist strings are worn to prevent soul loss—a state that resolves in illness. Infants may wear the strings around the neck, ankles, or waist. Emotional disturbances may manifest somatically because shame is connected to mental illness in this culture. Speaking loudly, yelling, snapping fingers under the nose, pointing, beckoning with finger, or hand outstretched with palm up offends others. Women officially use their husband's last name, and names are written in the following order: family name, middle name, and given name. The woman's lower torso is extremely private; the area between waist and knees is kept covered.

BIBLIOGRAPHY

Crow GK: Toward a theory of therapeutic syncretism: the Southeast Asian experience: a study of the Cambodians' use of traditional and cosmopolitan health systems, Doctoral dissertation, Salt Lake City, 1988, University of Utah.

Frye BA: The process of health care decision making among Cambodian immigrant women, *Appl Res Eval* 10(2):113, 1989-1990.

Frye BA: The Cambodian refugee patient: providing culturally sensitive rehabilitation nursing care, *Rehab Nurs* 15(3):156, 1990.

Frye BA: Cultural themes in health-care decision-making among Cambodian refugee women, *J Community Health Nurs* 8(1):33, 1991.

Galanti GA: *Caring for patients from different cultures,* Philadelphia, 1991, University of Pennsylvania Press.

Kulig JC: Contraception and birth control use: Cambodian refugee women's beliefs and practices, *J Community Health Nurs* 5(4):235, 1988.

Lawson LV: Culturally sensitive support for grieving parents, *MCN* 15:76, 1990.

Lenart JC, St. Clair PA, Bell MA: Childrearing knowledge, beliefs, and practices of Cambodian refugees, *J Pediatr Health Care* 5(6):299, 1991.

Li GR: *Funeral practices,* New York, World Relief, n.d.

Muecke MA: Caring for Southeast Asian refugee patients in the USA, *Am J Pub Health* 73(4):431, 1983.

Nguyen A, Bounthinh T, Mum S: *Folk medicine, folk nutrition, superstitions,* Washington, DC, 1980, Team Associates.

Rosenberg J: Cambodian children integrating treatment plans, *Pediatr Nurse* 12:118, 1986.

Schreiner D: S.E. *Asian folk healing practices-child abuse?* Eugene, Ore, 1981, Indochinese Health Care Conference.

Stewart EC, Bennett MJ: *American cultural patterns: a cross-cultural perspective,* rev ed, Yarmouth, Me, 1991, Intercultural Press.

Uland E, Smith S: Southeast Asian mental health issues, unpublished manuscript, 1984.

U.S. Department of Health, Education, and Welfare Social Security

Administration Office of Family Assistance, SSA 77-21013: *A guide to two cultures: Indochinese,* Washington DC, n.d.

Vandeusen J et al: South East Asian social and cultural customs: similarities and differences, *J Refugee Resettlement* 1:20, 1980.

◆ CAMEROON

MAP PAGE (260)

Location: Cameroon is a West African nation with a high plateau in the interior and swamps and plains along the coast of the Gulf of Guinea. English and French are the official languages, with over 200 vernacular languages spoken.

Major Languages	Ethnic Groups		Major Religions	
English	Cameroon		Indigenous	
French	Highlander	31%	Beliefs	51%
African Lan-	Equatorial		Christian	33%
guages	Bantu	19%	Muslim	16%
	Kirdi	11%		
	Fulani	10%		
	N.W. Bantu			
	and Other	29%		

Predominant Sick Care Practices: Biomedical; magico-religious.

Health Care Beliefs: Passive role; acute sick care. A primary health care policy was enacted in 1982; however, the people and the majority of health care practitioners still operate on a curative model.

Ethnic/Race Specific or Endemic Diseases: ENDEMIC: Yellow fever; chloroquine-resistant malaria. RISK: Cholera; schistosomiasis; intestinal parasites; diarrhea.

Families' Role in Hospital Care: Relatives provide routine bedside care for hospitalized patients.

National Childhood Immunizations: BCG at birth; DPT-1 at 2 months; DPT-2 at 3 months; DPT-3 at 4 months; DPT booster 1 year after DPT-3; measles at 9 months; OPV at birth; OPV-1 at 2 months; OPV-2 at 3 months; OPV-3 at 4 months; OPV booster 1 year after OPV-3.

BIBLIOGRAPHY

Awasum HM: Health and nursing services in Cameroon: challenges and demands for nurses in leadership positions, *Nurs Admin Q* 16(2):8, 1992.

Jato MN: Teaching future nursing teachers primary health care, *Int Nurs Rev* 29(6):189, 1982.

Jato MN et al: Community participation in rural health care, *Int Nurs Rev* 31(6):180, 1984.

◆ CAPE VERDE

MAP PAGE (260)

Location: These mountainous Atlantic Islands are 385 miles (620 km) off the coast of Senegal in Africa.

Major Languages	Ethnic Groups		Major Religions	
Portuguese	Creole	71%	Catholic	65%
Crioulo	African	28%	Indigenous	
	European	1%	Beliefs	35%

Predominant Sick Care Practices: Biomedical; traditional. Mixing traditional beliefs and modern concepts, Cape Verdeans believe that illness may be caused by neglecting social norms; therefore healthy people may seek medical care because they may be causing a family member's disease. The "patient" may never mention these family-related problems.

Ethnic/Race Specific or Endemic Diseases: ENDEMIC: Chloroquine-sensitive malaria; yellow fever.

Infant Feeding Practices: A belief exists that after delivery, sexual contact with a man other than the newborn's father results in a mixing of the adults' blood, poisoning the mother's milk. The poison's effect on the infant may be delayed.

National Childhood Immunizations: BCG at birth; DPT-1 at 6 weeks; DPT-2 at 10 weeks; DPT-3 at 14 weeks; DPT booster 1 year after DPT-3; measles at 9 months; OPV at birth; OPV-1 at 6 weeks; OPV-2 at 10 weeks; OPV-3 at 14 weeks; OPV booster 1 year after OPV-3.

BIBLIOGRAPHY

Reitmaier P: The death of Amilcar: a case study from Santo Antao/Cabo Verde, *Ann Soc Belg Med Trop* 67(suppl 1):111, 1987.

◆ CENTRAL AFRICAN REPUBLIC

MAP PAGE (260)

Location: A landlocked republic 500 miles (805 km) north of the African equator, the country is covered with tropical forest in the south and with semidesert land in the east. It is one of the 25 poorest countries in the world.

Major Languages	Ethnic Groups		Major Religions	
French	Baya	34%	Protestant	25%
Sangho	Banda	27%	Catholic	25%
Arabic	Mandjia	21%	Indigenous	
Hunsa	Sara	10%	Beliefs	24%
Swahili	Mboum and		Muslim	26%
	Other	8%		

Ethnic/Race Specific or Endemic Diseases: ENDEMIC: Chloroquine-resistant malaria; yellow fever. **RISK:** Schistosomiasis. AIDS case rate is 23.1/100,000 people.

National Childhood Immunizations: BCG at birth; DPT-1 at 6 weeks; DPT-2 at 10 weeks; DPT-3 at 14 weeks; DPT booster at 16 months; measles at 9 months; yellow fever at 1 year; OPV at birth; OPV-1 at 6 weeks; OPV-2 at 10 weeks; OPV-3 at 14 weeks; OPV booster at 16 months.

BIBLIOGRAPHY

Adler MW, editor: Statistics from the World Health Organization and the Centers for Disease Control, *AIDS* 6(10):1229, 1992.

◆ CHAD

MAP PAGE (260)

Location: Chad is a landlocked country in north central Africa, with a northern desert that runs into the Sahara. Chad is one of the poorest countries in the world; most of its population live in poverty and are without easy access to safe water and basic sanitation facilities. Most of its 186 miles (300 km) of paved roads are impassable during and after the rainy season (June through September).

Major Languages	Ethnic Groups		Major Religions	
French	Muslim		Muslim	44%
Arabic	Groups	44%	Christian	33%
Sara	Non-Muslim		Indigenous	
Sango	Groups	25%	Beliefs	23%
Other	Other	31%		

Ethnic/Race Specific or Endemic Diseases: ENDEMIC: Yellow fever; schistosomiasis; chloroquine-resistant malaria. RISK: Cholera.

Death Rites: For Muslim burial, the body is wrapped in special pieces of cloth and buried without a coffin in the ground. Cremation is not permitted.

National Childhood Immunizations: BCG at birth; DPT-1 at 6 weeks; DPT-2 at 10 weeks; DPT-3 at 14 weeks; yellow fever at 6 months; measles at 9 months; OPV at birth; OPV-1 at 6 weeks; OPV-2 at 10 weeks; OPV-3 at 14 weeks.

BIBLIOGRAPHY

Ross HM: Societal/cultural views regarding death and dying, *Top Clin Nurs* 1(1):1, 1981.

Stiegler KS: All-out effort thwarts Chad cholera crisis, *Front Lines* 31(11):10, 1991.

◆ CHILE

MAP PAGE (258)

Location: The country fills a narrow 1800-mile-strip (2897 km) between the Andes mountains and the Pacific Ocean. One third of Chile is covered by towering mountain ranges; the southernmost city in the world is located at its tip. A 700-mile (1127 km) valley in the center is thickly populated; in the north is the Atacama desert.

Major Language	Ethnic Groups		Major Religions	
Spanish	European and		Catholic	89%
	Mestizo	95%	Protestant	
	Native		and	
	American	3%	Other	11%
	Other	2%		

Health Care Beliefs: Acute sick care only.

Ethnic/Race Specific or Endemic Diseases: RISK: Malnutrition in poorer areas.

Birth Rites: Use of contraceptives is limited. Rhythm is a popular birth control practice. Many believe that a woman should have as many children as God gives her. Abortion is illegal.

National Childhood Immunizations: DPT-1 at 2 months; DPT-2 at 4 months; DPT-3 at 6 months; DPT boosters at 18 months and 4 years; OPV-1 at 2 months; OPV-2 at 4 months; OPV-3 at 6 months; OPV boosters at 18 months and 4 years; measles at 12 months; BCG at birth.

BIBLIOGRAPHY

Anderson F: Chilean midwifery: under the jackboot, *Nurs Times* 85(31):74, 1989.

Burkhalter BR, Marin PS: A demonstration of increased exclusive breastfeeding in Chile, *Int J Gynaecol Obstet* 34(4):353, 1991.

Perez A, Valdes V: Santiago breastfeeding promotion program: preliminary results of an intervention study, *Am J Obstet Gynecol* 165 Part 2:2039, 1991.

Scarpaci JL: Help-seeking behavior, use, and satisfaction among frequent primary care users in Santiago de Chile, *J Health Soc Behav* 29(3):199, 1988.

Valenzuela MS et al: Survey of reproductive health in young adults, Greater Santiago, *Bull Pan Am Health Org* 25(4):293, 1991.

◆ CHINA

MAP PAGE (263)

Location: The world's third largest country, China, occupies the eastern part of Asia. Western China is mountainous, arid, and isolated; the eastern third has fertile agricultural land and river deltas. Tibet and Taiwan are part of the Republic of China; however, Taiwan is currently not subject to Mainland China.

Major Languages	Ethnic Groups		Major Religions	
Mandarin	Han Chinese	94%	Atheist and	
Cantonese	Other	6%	Eclectic	97%
Shanghainese			Other	3%
Fuzhou				
Minnan and				
Other				

Predominant Sick Care Practices: Holistic; traditional. Chinese medicine is one of the oldest practiced in the world, with a theoretical base and diagnostic and treatment modalities still in use today. Traditional health care includes moxibustion (cupping), acupuncture, and herbal medicine.

Health Care Beliefs: Health promotion is important. The Chinese are the first to attribute an upset in body energy to the cause of disease. Health is believed to be a state of spiritual and physical harmony with nature; health and illness are not separate but part of a lifelong continuum. Some resist surgery because of a religious belief that they do not own their physical bodies, that the soul or spirit will escape from the body and be lost forever if surgery is performed. Drawing blood may be resisted because of the belief that blood does not regenerate; blood is perceived as the source of life. Taking medications while feeling well is an alien concept to some Chinese. Stigma is attached to mental illness; therefore severe personality disorganization is the only criterion for entering the health care system.

Ethnic/Race Specific or Endemic Diseases: ENDEMIC: Chloroquine-sensitive; resistant malaria. RISK: Japanese encephalitis; schistosomiasis; adult lactase deficiency; alpha thalassemia; Chinese-type G6PD deficiency; viral hepatitis. Neurasthenia (nerve exhaustion) is a common modern Chinese psychiatric disorder; psychological symptoms include anxiety states, depression, and hypochondria. Hypertension, diabetes, and cancer are the leading causes of death.

Health Team Relationships: Most nurses are female. Male nurses usually work in urology or psychiatric services. Nurses serve in supplementary roles to physicians, and social assertiveness is not emphasized. Nurses and physicians are authority figures or experts, and patients are not given much information about their illnesses, medicines, or diagnostic procedures. Patients do not express their concerns about prescribed interventions or treatments. Thoughts are expressed politely and with restraint through language that is indirect. The listener is expected to understand. Physicians rely heavily on inspection and palpation in making diagnoses.

Families' Role in Hospital Care: A family member may be given leave from work to care for an aged relative. The family traditionally remains with the patient during hospitalization, supplying food and assisting with feeding, bathing, and keeping the patient comfortable.

Dominance Patterns: The family unit is more important than the individual. Marked role differentiation is based on age, gender, and generation. The aged are not segregated and have high status. Older Chinese parents take pride in being supported and cared for by their children. Father/son relationships are strong. Devotion to parents includes caring for them physically and psychologically. In decision-making, the young defer to the old; both parents make decisions concerning the child.

Eye Contact Practices: Gazing around and looking to one side when listening to another are polite. With the elderly, however, direct eye contact is used.

Touch Practices: Chinese do not like to be touched by strangers. Introductions elicit a nod or a slight bow.

Perceptions of Time: An inexact, patient, and broad orientation is taken toward time. The past is valued, and traditional approaches to healing are preferred over new procedures or medications. Recently, China seems to be shifting to a more futuristic orientation.

Pain Reactions: Strong negative feelings, such as anger and pain, are often suppressed. A display of emotion is considered a weakness of character. Because it is considered impolite to accept something the first time it is offered, pain relief interventions must be offered more than once.

Birth Rites: Amniocentesis may be used to determine the sex of a fetus. The government limitation of one child per family causes some to consider abortion if the fetus is female. Premature birth weight is suggested at 2300 g. Fathers are not seen in labor rooms, delivery rooms, or postpartum areas. Women labor fully clothed and deliver in the low lithotomy position. Acupuncture is used during labor induction, stimulation, and Caesarean section. After childbirth the mother is separated from her baby for 12 to 24 hours and does not bathe for 7 to 30 days; she is permitted to eat only certain foods. Keeping warm is important. Mothers with one child use IUDs. National regulations forbid removal of the birth control device. The newborn is considered 1 year old at birth.

Death Rites: The Chinese have an aversion to death and to anything concerning death. Autopsy and disposal of the body are individual preferences and are not prescribed by religion. Euthanasia is permitted, and donation of body parts is encouraged. The eldest son is responsible for all arrangements for the deceased. The deceased is initially buried in a coffin. After 7 years, the body is exhumed and cremated, and the urn is reburied in a tomb. White clothing is worn as a sign of mourning.

Food Practices and Intolerances: The diet is low in fat. Excessive amounts of soy sauce and dried and preserved foods contribute to high sodium intake. Herbs are used to treat symptoms, wounds, and disease. The ginseng root is widely used. Raw vegetables and meats are usually not eaten. Hot and warm beverages are preferred.

Infant Feeding Practices: Breastfeeding is encouraged and may be continued for 4 to 5 years. Cow milk and goat milk are not acceptable alternatives for breastmilk.

Child Rearing Practices: Young children are reared in a permissive environment but are constantly cared for. When the child is old enough, repressive authority is encountered; the child is expected to develop self-control. Until school age, children are placed in a day care facility or with family elders. Children are taught to show respect and deference to parents and authority figures. To discipline, the parents shame the children or make them feel guilty. These tactics may be followed by reasoning. Children learn to control their emotions; aggressive behavior is undesired and suppressed. Child abuse is rare. Children are taught to be unselfish and to function competitively in a group. Fathers are less involved in child rearing than are mothers. Mother/son relationships are close and long lived. In education, students are not free to choose their professions but are placed where the government believes they can best serve the nation.

National Childhood Immunizations: DPT at 3 months, 4 months, and 5 months; DPT booster at 1 year; school entry D or DT/DP varies based on local conditions in the provinces; polio at 2 months, 3 months, and 4 months; boosters at 1 year, 2 years, and 7 years; BCG at birth and 7 years; measles at 8 months.

Other Characteristics: The belief that illness needs to be drawn out of the body is practiced through coin rubbing. A heated coin or one smeared with oil is vigorously rubbed over the body, producing red welts. It is believed that the red welts will only occur if people are ill.

BIBLIOGRAPHY

Bowling SK: International psychiatric nursing delegates: a visit to China, *Kansas Nurse* 66(4):14, 1991.

Boyle JS, Andrews MM: *Transcultural concepts in nursing care,* Glenview, Ill, 1989, Scott, Foresman/Little, Brown College Division.

Breiner SJ: Early child development in China, *Child Psychiatry Hum Dev* 11(2):87, 1980.

Brower HT: Culture and nursing in China, *Nurs Health Care* 5(1):27, 1984.

Brown BS: Growing up healthy, the Chinese experience, *Pediatr Nurs* 9(4):255, 1983.

Chae M: Older Asians, *J Gerontol Nurs* 13(11):11, 1987.

Chinese revolutions—health care overseas, *Nurs Times* 85(29):48, 1989.

Condon JC, Yousef F: *An introduction to intercultural communication,* New York, 1975, Macmillan.

DeSantis L: Bridging the gap: cultural diversity in nursing. Paper presented to the Florida Nurses Association, 1990.

Dirschel KM: International nursing exchange: the United States and China, *Perspectives in nursing—1985-1987,* New York, 1985, National League for Nursing.

Discovery Channel: A planet for the taking, March 15, 1989.

Dollar B: *The child care in China.* In Wurzel JS, editor: *Toward multiculturalism: a reader in multicultural education,* Yarmouth, Me, 1988, Intercultural Press.

Duncan L: Contributor.

Eisenbruch M: Cross-cultural aspects of bereavement, Part 2, Ethnic and cultural variations in the development of bereavement practices, *Cult Med Psychol* 8(4):315, 1984.

Ekblad S: Social determinants of aggression in a sample of Chinese primary school children, *Acta Psychiatry Scand* 73(5):515, 1986.

Ekblad S: Influence of child-rearing on aggressive behavior in a transcultural perspective, *Acta Psychiatr Scand Suppl* 344:133, 1988.

Elder SP, Hsia L: Women's health care and the workplace and the People's Republic of China, *J Nurse-Midwifery* 31(4):182, 1986.

Farb P: *Man at the mercy of language.* In Wurzel JS, editor: *Toward multiculturalism: a reader in multicultural education,* Yarmouth, Me, 1988, Intercultural Press.

Fisher P: Chinese population crises. Paper submitted for Sociology 107W, Storrs, 1989, University of Connecticut.

Galanti GA: *Caring for patients from different cultures,* Philadelphia, 1991, University of Pennsylvania Press.

Greenhalgh S, Bongaarts J: Fertility policy in China: future options, *Science* 235:1167, 1987.

Holtzen VL: A comparative study of nursing in China and the United States, *Nurs Forum* 22(3):86, 1985.

Horn BM: Cultural concepts and postpartal care, *Nurs Health Care* 2(9):516, 1981.

Hsiao WC: Transformation of health care in China, *N Engl J Med* 310(14):932, 1984.

Human rights in China, *Beijing Review* 34(44):8, 1991.

Iorio J, Nelson MA: China: caring's the same, *Nurs Outlook* 31(2):100, 1983.

Jung M: Structural family therapy: its application to Chinese families, *Fam Proc* 23(3):365, 1984.

Kong DS et al: Child-rearing practices of Chinese parents and their relationship to behavioural problems in toddlers, *Acta Psychiatr Scand Suppl* 344:127, 1988.

Liu YC: China: health care in transition, *Nurs Outlook* 31(2):94, 1983.

Lockhart JD: The children of China, *Hosp Pract* 14(2):118, 1979.

Martinelli AM: Pain and ethnicity: how people of different cultures experience pain, *AORN J* 46(2):273, 1987.

McKay S: Maternity care in China: report of a tour of Chinese medical facilities, *Birth* 9(2):105, 1982.

Morrisey S: Attitudes on aging in China, *J Gerontol Nurs* 9(11):589, 1983.

Muecke MA: Caring for Southeast Asian refugee patients in the USA, *Am J Pub Health* 73(4):431, 1983.

Overfield T: *Biologic variation in health and illness,* Menlo Park, Calif, 1985, Addison-Wesley.

Prosser MH: *The cultural dialogue,* Washington, DC, 1985, SIETAR.

Randolph G: The Yin and Yang of clinical practice, *Top Clin Nurs* 1(1):31, 1979.

Sawyer F: ABC News, June 2, 1991.

Spector RE: *Cultural diversity in health and illness,* ed 3, Norwalk, Conn, 1991, Appleton & Lange.

Stewart EC, Bennett MJ: *American cultural patterns: a cross-cultural perspective,* rev ed, Yarmouth, Me, 1991, Intercultural Press.

Teeng WS et al: Family planning and child mental health in China: the Nanjing survey, *Am J Psychiatry* 145(11):1396, 1988.

Tien-Hyatt JL: Keying in on the unique care needs of Asian clients, *Nurs Health Care* 8(5):269, 1987.

Tseng V, Hsu J: The Chinese attitude toward parental authority as expressed in Chinese children's stories, *Arch Gen Psychiatry* 26(1):28, 1972.

Xiangdong M, Blum RW: School health services in the People's Republic of China, *J School Health* 60(10):483, 1990.

Zhan L: Guest lecture, NURS 285, Storrs, 1991, University of Connecticut.

◆ COLOMBIA

MAP PAGE (258)

Location: Colombia is the only country in South America that borders the Atlantic and the Pacific Oceans. It is composed of low coastal plains along the oceans and three parallel mountain ranges: the Andes, running north to south. The climate is dependent on altitude. At the end of the 1980s about one fifth of the population lived in poverty.

Major Languages	Ethnic Groups		Major Religions	
Spanish	Mestizo	58%	Catholic	95%
Indian dialects	White	28%	Other	5%
	Mulatto	14%		
	African	4%		
	Native American and Other	4%		

Predominant Sick Care Practices: Biomedical; magico-religious. The Mestizo believe that people are controlled by environment, that nature can be dangerous, and that nature is animated by the presence of spirits.

Ethnic/Race Specific or Endemic Diseases: ENDEMIC: Chloroquine-resistant malaria. RISK: Yellow fever; dengue fever; cholera; mild protein deficiency malnutrition; iron deficiency anemia.

Touch Practices: Touch is important, and hugs are used in greeting others.

Perceptions of Time: Relaxed.

Birth Rites: Traditional Catholics believe that abortion is a sin. If the father is consulted, his decision about continuing or terminating the pregnancy is usually followed. Significant numbers of women use contraceptives; however, sterilization is preferred.

Food Practices and Intolerances: The main meal is in late evening.

National Childhood Immunizations: DPT-1 at 2 months; DPT-2 at 4 months; DPT-3 at 6 months; OPV-1 at 2 months; OPV-2 at 4 months; OPV-3 at 6 months; measles at 9 months; BCG at birth.

Other Characteristics: Injections of oil are used to treat infections and cause hard lumps under the skin. To indicate a person's height by extending the arm with the palm down is an insulting gesture. The city of Bogota created international interest in their system of Kangaroo Care for treatment of premature (low birth weight) infants.

BIBLIOGRAPHY

Anderson GC, Marks E, Wahlberg V: Kangaroo care for premature infants, *AJN* 86(7):807, 1986.

Browner C: *The role of faculty development in multicultural education,* Los Angeles, Prism Publishing of Mount St. Mary's College, no date provided.

de Prjuela ML: Evolution of nursing: its influence and commitment in the social development of Colombia, *J Prof Nurs* 5(6):330, 1989.

Geissler EM: Personal journal, 1967.

Hollerbach P: The impact of national policies on the acceptance of sterilization in Colombia and Costa Rica, *Stud Fam Plan* 20(6):308, 1989.

Irujo S: *An introduction to intercultural differences and similarities in nonverbal communication.* In Wurzel JS, editor: *Toward multiculturalism,* Yarmouth, Me, 1988, Intercultural Press.

Stewart EC, Bennett MJ: *American cultural patterns: a cross-cultural perspective,* rev ed, Yarmouth, Me, 1991, Intercultural Press.

Virgin C, Jacobsen U: More female warmth and less high technology. Paper presented at the Fifth International Council on Women's Health Issues, 1992, Copenhagen.

World Monitor TV: April 11, 1991.

◆ COMOROS

MAP PAGE (261)

Location: The three volcanic islands of Comoros (Grande Comoro, Anjouan, and Moheli) are located in the Mozambique Channel of the Indian Ocean between Madagascar and Africa.

Major Languages	Ethnic Groups		Major Religions	
Shaafi Islam	Arab	40%	Sunni	
Malagasy	African	38%	Muslim	86%
French	East Indian		Catholic	14%
	and Other	22%		

Ethnic/Race Specific or Endemic Diseases: ENDEMIC: Chloroquine-resistant malaria.

Death Rites: The Muslim belief forbids organ donation or transplants. Muslim physicians may recommend transfusions to save lives. Autopsy is uncommon because the deceased must be buried intact. Cremation is not permitted. For Muslim burial the body is wrapped in special pieces of cloth and buried without a coffin in the ground.

National Childhood Immunizations: BCG at birth; DPT-1 at 6 weeks; DPT-2 at 10 weeks; DPT-3 at 14 weeks; DPT booster 1 year after DPT-3; measles at 9 months; OPV-1 at 6 weeks; OPV-2 at 10 weeks; OPV-3 at 14 weeks; OPV booster 1 year after OPV-3.

BIBLIOGRAPHY

Ross HM: Societal/cultural views regarding death and dying, *Top Clin Nurs* 1(1):1, 1981.

♦ CONGO

MAP PAGE (261)

Location: This west central African nation (formerly the French Congo) lies astride the equator. It is covered by thick tropical rain forests.

Major Languages	Ethnic Groups		Major Religions	
French	Kongo	48%	Christian	50%
Lingala	Sangha	20%	Animist	42%
Kikongo	Teke	17%	Muslim	2%
Other	M'Bochi	12%	Other	6%
	Other	3%		

Ethnic/Race Specific or Endemic Diseases: ENDEMIC: Yellow fever; chloroquine-resistant malaria. RISK: Schistosomiasis, Crimean-Congo hemorrhagic fever. AIDS case rate is 20.5/100,000 people.

National Childhood Immunizations: BCG at birth; DPT-1 at 2 months; DPT-2 at 3 months; DPT-3 at 4 months; measles at 9 months; OPV at birth; OPV-1 at 2 months; OPV-2 at 3 months; OPV-3 at 4 months.

BIBLIOGRAPHY

Adler MW, editor: Statistics from the World Health Organization and the Centers for Disease Control, *AIDS* 6(10):1229, 1992.

Paverd N: Crimean-Congo haemorrhagic fever: a nursing care plan, *Nurs Rsa Verpleging* 3(4):33, 1988.

Paverd N: Crimean-Congo haemorrhagic fever: a protocol for control and containment in a health care facility, *Nurs Rsa Verpleging* 3(7):33, 1988.

◆ COSTA RICA

MAP PAGE (256)

Location: Costa Rica spans the width of a narrow section of Central America in the tropical zone. Most people live at the higher temperate altitudes. This country has one of the lowest death rates in the world and has achieved a relatively high standard of living and social services.

Major Languages	Ethnic Groups		Major Religions	
Spanish	European	96%	Catholic	95%
Creole	Black	3%	Other	5%
	Native			
	American	1%		

Predominant Sick Care Practices: Biomedical; magico-religious; traditional. The people frequently use traditional medicinal plants (bush medicines) along with over-the-counter Western medicines. Some believe that one type of medicine cannot cure many different diseases.

Health Care Beliefs: Health promotion is important. State-of-health population indicators are similar to those of developed nations. The hot/cold theory and keeping the body in balance promote preventive health care.

Ethnic/Race Specific or Endemic Diseases: RISK: Chloroquine-sensitive malaria; parasite infestation; malnutrition.

Touch Practices: Costa Ricans touch frequently.

Child Rearing Practices: In 1982 contraception by sterilization was rendered illegal.

National Childhood Immunizations: DPT-1 at 2 months; DPT-2 at 4 months; DPT-3 at 6 months; DPT boosters at 18 months and 4 years; OPV-1 at 2 months; OPV-2 at 4 months; OPV-3 at 6 months; OPV boosters at 18 months and 4 years; measles at 12 months; BCG at birth, and, if warranted, at 7 and 12 years.

BIBLIOGRAPHY

Giger JN, Davidhizar RE: *Transcultural nursing,* St Louis, 1991, Mosby.
Hill CE: Local health knowledge and universal primary health care: a behavioral case from Costa Rica, *Med Anthropol* 9(1):11, 1985.
Hollerbach P: The impact of national policies on the acceptance of sterilization in Colombia and Costa Rica, *Stud Fam Plan* 20(6):308, 1989.
Mohs E: General theory of paradigms in health, *Scand J Soc Med Suppl* 46:14, 1991.

◆ CUBA

MAP PAGE (257)

Location: Cuba, the largest and westernmost island of the West Indies, is located 90 miles (145 km) south of the southern tip of Florida.

Major Language	Ethnic Groups		Major Religions	
Spanish	Mulatto	51%	Catholic	85%
	White	37%	Other	15%
	Black	11%		
	Chinese	1%		

Predominant Sick Care Practices: Biomedical; magico-religious. Santeria is a blend of African and Catholic religions and health care beliefs.

Health Care Beliefs: Active involvement; health promotion important. Supernatural forces (evil eye) is thought to cause some illnesses that must be cured by ethnic treatments or magic spells. Amulets on a bracelet or necklace or pinned to clothing provide some protection against the evil eye. Illness prevention and health promotion programs and facilities are in place nationwide.

Ethnic/Race Specific or Endemic Diseases: Polio, malaria, and diphtheria have been eradicated.

Health Team Relationships: Physicians and nurses visit the homes of the ill. Such programs strengthen relationships between the health care professionals and the community.

Families' Role in Hospital Care: Parents can stay overnight and give personal care to hospitalized children.

Death Rites: Family and friends remain with the deceased through the night. Burial is within 24 hours. After the burial, family and friends stay up for 9 consecutive days; the less traditional replace this with a holy hour each evening.

Food Practices and Intolerances: The adult diet tends to be high in fat, cholesterol, sugar, and fried foods.

Infant Feeding Practices: Traditionally, plump babies and young children are idealized.

Child Rearing Practices: The mother explains and reasons as she rears her child. These methods anticipate and prepare the child for developmental tasks. Mothers or parents should be included in health education programs. The school system provides health teaching and assumes much of the child-rearing responsibilities.

National Childhood Immunizations: DPT-1 at 3 months; DPT-2 at 4 months; DPT-3 at 5 months; DPT booster at 18 months; OPV-1 at 1 month; OPV-2 at 3 months; OPV-3 at 1 year; OPV boosters at 2, 3, 4, and 9 years; measles at

9 months and 6 years; BCG, if warranted, at birth and 10 years.

BIBLIOGRAPHY

DeSantis L, Thomas, JT: Parental attitudes toward adolescent sexuality: transcultural perspectives, *Nurs Pract* 12(8):43, 1987.

Guttmacher S: The prevention of health risks in Cuba, *Int J Health Serv* 17(1):179, 1987.

Guttmacher S: Minimizing health risks in Cuba, *Med Anthropol* 11:167, 1989.

Li GR: *Funeral practices,* New York, World Relief, n.d.

Martinson IM et al: The block nurse program, *J Commun Health Nurs* 2(1):21, 1985.

Pasquali E: Santeria: a religion and health care system for Long Island Cuban-Americans, *Cultural Connections* 7(3):1, 1987.

Ruiz P: Cultural barriers to effective medical care among Hispanic-American patients, *Annu Rev Med* 36:63, 1985.

Swanson JM: Nursing in Cuba: population-focused practice, *Pub Health Nurs* 4(3):183, 1987.

Swanson JM: Health-care delivery in Cuba: nursing's role in achievement of the goal of "Health for All," *Int J Nurs Stud* 25(1):11, 1988.

◆ CYPRUS

MAP PAGE (262)

Location: Cyprus is a Mediterranean island off the southern coast of Turkey; it has a broad central plain between mountain ranges.

Major Languages	Ethnic Groups		Major Religions	
Greek	Greek	78%	Greek	
Turkish	Turkish	18%	Orthodox	78%
English	Armenian		Muslim	18%
	and Other	4%	Other	4%

National Childhood Immunizations: OPV-1 at 3 months; OPV-2 at 5 months; OPV-3 at 7 months.

BIBLIOGRAPHY

Angel JL: Genetic and social factors in a Cypriote village, *Hum Biol* 44(1):53, 1972.

Volkan VD: Mourning and adaptation after a war, *Am J Psychother* 31(4):561, 1977.

◆ CZECHOSLOVAKIA

MAP PAGE (258)

Location: This landlocked, mountainous country is located in central Europe.

Major Languages	Ethnic Groups		Major Religions	
Czech	Czech	64%	Catholic	77%
Slovak	Slovak	31%	Protestant	20%
Hungarian	Hungarian	4%	Orthodox	2%
	German		Other	1%
	and Other	1%		

Child Rearing Practices: Dependency, security, obligation, and reciprocity within the extended family are valued.

National Childhood Immunizations: BCG at 4-6 weeks; OPV at birth, 15 weeks, and 13 years; DPT at 9 weeks, 15 weeks, and between 3 and 6 months; measles at 15 months; measles and rubella between 21 and 25 months; rubella for girls at 12 years.

BIBLIOGRAPHY

Stein F: The Slovak-American swaddling ethos: homeostate for family dynamics and cultural continuity, *Fam Proc* 17(1):31, 1978.
Utley G: NBC-TV Nightly News, July 19, 1992.

◆ DENMARK

MAP PAGE (258)

Location: Denmark is situated on the Jutland Peninsula and on neighboring islands that separate the North and

Baltic seas in northern Europe. It is the smallest and flattest of the Scandinavian countries. Its highest point is 570 feet (174 m) above sea level.

Major Languages	Ethnic Groups		Major Religions	
Danish	Danish	99%	Lutheran	97%
Faroese	Other	1%	Other Christian	2%
			Other	1%

Predominant Sick Care Practices: Biomedical; magico-religious; and traditional.

Health Care Beliefs: Active involvement; passive role; health promotion important.

Ethnic/Race Specific or Endemic Diseases: RISK: Krabbe disease; phenylketonuria.

Health Team Relationships: Collegial relationships may exist among nurses and physicians, or physicians may expect nurses to fulfill service roles.

Families' Role in Hospital Care: Nurses provide all patient care; however, families may help with children.

Dominance Patterns: Some males have a slight dominant edge.

Eye Contact Practices: Direct eye contact is expected and is held.

Touch Practices: Touching is infrequent and is used with friends and associates only.

Perceptions of Time: Promptness is valued.

Pain Reactions: Patients are willing to inform the health care professional that they are in pain.

Food Practices and Intolerances: Breakfast may consist of combinations of yogurt products, white bread, coffee, corn flakes, cheese, and orange juice. The largest meal is taken between 6 and 8 PM. Spaghetti is currently a popular food among young people.

Infant Feeding Practices: Breastfeeding is most common.

National Childhood Immunizations: Pertussis at 5 weeks, 9 weeks, and 10 months; DT at 5 months, 6 months, and

15 months; MMR at 15 months and 12 years; injectable polio at 5 months, 6 months, and 15 months; OPV at 2 years, 3 years, and 4 years.

Other Characteristics: During conversation, periods of silence are valued.

BIBLIOGRAPHY

Boyle JS, Andrews MM: *Transcultural concepts in nursing care,* Glenview, Ill, 1989, Scott, Foresman/Little, Brown College Division.

Geissler EM: Personal observations and communications, August 22-29, 1992.

Larsen AS: Helping patients avoid readmission to hospital: a health behaviour study, *Recent Adv Nurs* 22:62, 1988.

Lindquist GJ: Primary health care in four countries, *J Prof Nurs* 2(4):203, 1986.

Menyuk P, Menyuk D: *Communicative competence: a historical and cultural perspective.* In Wurzel JS: *Toward multiculturalism,* Yarmouth, Me, 1988, Intercultural Press.

Merrick J: Physical punishment of children in Denmark: an historical perspective, *Child Abuse Negl* 10(2):263, 1986.

Wagner L: A proposed model for care of the elderly, *Int Nurs Rev* 36(2):50, 1989.

◆ DJIBOUTI

MAP PAGE (260)

Location: Formerly French Somaliland (from 1967 to 1977 the Territory of the Afars and Issus), this sparsely populated, small country lies in Northeast Africa at the southern entrance to the Red Sea. The area is arid, sandy, and desolate.

Major Languages	Ethnic Groups		Major Religions	
French	Somali Issa	60%	Muslim	94%
Arabic	Afar	35%	Christian	6%
Issa	Other	5%		
Afar				

Ethnic/Race Specific or Endemic Diseases: ENDEMIC: Yellow fever; chloroquine-sensitive malaria. AIDS case rate is 12.5/100,000 people.

Death Rites: Muslim belief forbids organ donation or transplants. Muslim physicians may recommend transfusions to save lives. Autopsy is uncommon because the deceased must be buried intact. Cremation is not permitted. For Muslim burial the body is wrapped in special pieces of cloth and buried without a coffin in the ground.

National Childhood Immunizations: OPV-1 at 3 months; OPV-2 at 4 months; OPV-3 at 5 months.

BIBLIOGRAPHY

Adler MW, editor: Statistics from the World Health Organization and the Centers for Disease Control, *AIDS* 6(10):1229, 1992.

Ross HM: Societal/cultural views regarding death and dying, *Top Clin Nurs* 1(1):1, 1981.

◆ DOMINICA

MAP PAGE (257)

Location: An eastern Caribbean island discovered by Columbus in 1493.

Major Languages	Ethnic Groups		Major Religions	
English	Black	98%	Catholic	80%
French Patois	Other	2%	Protestant	20%

BIBLIOGRAPHY

No data located.

◆ DOMINICAN REPUBLIC

MAP PAGE (257)

Location: This country occupies the eastern two thirds of the Caribbean island of Hispaniola, sharing it with Haiti.

Major Language	Ethnic Groups		Major Religions	
Spanish	Mixed	73%	Catholic	95%
	White	16%	Other	5%
	Black	11%		

Predominant Sick Care Practices: Magico-religious; traditional.

Health Care Beliefs: The hot/cold balance theory is a factor in the cause of disease. (See Cambodia, p. 36.)

Ethnic/Race Specific or Endemic Diseases: ENDEMIC: Chloroquine-sensitive malaria below 400 m. RISK: Dengue; schistosomiasis.

Birth Rites: It is believed that cravings during pregnancy should be satisfied. Newborns may be kept indoors for a month. The traditional mother may not wish to bathe, wash her hair, or have intercourse for 40 days after giving birth. Protection of the child against the evil eye may take the form of wearing red clothing, and some may save the umbilical cord.

National Childhood Immunizations: Measles at 9 months; BCG at birth.

Other Characteristics: Anise tea is believed to have medicinal qualities.

BIBLIOGRAPHY

Nichols FH: Health status of children in rural areas of the Dominican Republic: policy implications for nursing practice and nursing education in Third World countries, *J Commun Health Nurs* 1(2):125, 1984.

Ruiz PM: Dominican concepts of health and illness, *J NY State Nurses Assoc* 21(4):11, 1990.

◆ ECUADOR

MAP PAGE (258)

Location: Ecuador is named for the equator, on which it lies. Two mountain ranges: the Andes, including the tall volcanic peaks (the highest, 20,577 feet [6272 m]), split the country into hot, humid lowlands on the Pacific coast. Temperate highlands are found between the ranges, as well as the mostly unexplored and uninhabited tropical jungle of the Amazon basin. The Galapagos Islands are part of the country.

Major Languages	Ethnic Groups		Major Religions	
Spanish	Mestizo	55%	Catholic	95%
Quechua	Native		Other	5%
English	American	25%		
German	Spanish	10%		
Jivaro	Black	10%		

Predominant Sick Care Practices: Traditional. A traditional healer is called a *brujo.*

Ethnic/Race Specific or Endemic Diseases: ENDEMIC: Yellow fever. RISK: Chloroquine-resistant malaria. ACTIVE: Cholera (in 1991); diarrheal disorders; protein-calorie malnutrition in children.

Dominance Patterns: The family's and an individual's position in society (rather than the family or individual) predominate. Several generations may live together, and the elderly are respected.

Touch Practices: It is acceptable for members of the same sex to touch, and men may greet one another with an embrace.

Perceptions of Time: Siesta time is during the afternoon.

Food Practices and Intolerances: Noon is the main meal. Staples include chicken, corn, potatoes, and beans. Fried foods are popular.

National Childhood Immunizations: DPT-1 at 3 months; DPT-2 at 6 months; DPT-3 at 9 months; DPT booster at 21 months; OPV-1 at 3 months; OPV-2 at 6 months; OPV-3 at 9 months; OPV booster at 21 months; measles at 9 months; BCG at birth and at 5 years.

BIBLIOGRAPHY

Axtell RE, editor: *Do's and taboos around the world,* ed 2, New York, 1990, John Wiley & Sons.

Finerman RD: A matter of life and death: health care change in an Andean community, *Soc Sci Med* 18(4):329, 1984.

Ruffing KL, Smith HL: Maternal and child health care in Ecuador: obstacles and solutions, *Health Care Women Int* 5(4):195, 1984.

Ruffing KL, Smith HL: Planning for rural community health nursing needs: the experience of Ecuador, *J Adv Nurs* 9(2):136, 1984.

Stewart EC, Bennett MJ: *American cultural patterns: a cross-cultural perspective,* rev ed, Yarmouth, Me, 1991, Intercultural Press.

World Monitor TV, April 11, 1991.

◆ EGYPT

MAP PAGE (260)

Location: Egypt occupies the northeast corner of Africa. Most of its citizens reside in the Nile river valley because 97% of Egypt is dry and arid desert.

Major Languages	Ethnic Groups		Major Religions	
Arabic	Eastern		Sunni	
English	Hamitic	90%	Muslim	94%
	Other	10%	Other	6%

Predominant Sick Care Practices: Biomedical; magico-religious. The evil eye, hot/cold disease factors (see Cambodia, p. 36.) are beliefs that coexist with Western medical practices.

Health Care Beliefs: Passive role. Injections and intravenous fluids are perceived as more effective. The belief that health is dictated by Allah promotes a passive role. Self-medication is practiced. Pharmacists and nurses can prescribe drugs. Amulets inscribed with verses of the Koran, turquoise stones, or a charm of a hand with five fingers enhance protective powers against the evil eye.

Ethnic/Race Specific or Endemic Diseases: ENDEMIC: Chloroquine-sensitive malaria. RISK: Schistosomiasis.

Health Team Relationships: The reason for asking personal questions during assessment needs to be clarified. Males may refuse care by female physicians or nurse practitioners, especially if the problem is a sexually sensitive one. Sudden termination of a long-term relationship between health care professional and patient is tactless and inconsiderate.

Families' Role in Hospital Care: Culture dictates that family and friends visit the patient as much as possible to ensure that health care personnel care for and attend the patient properly. Some may wish to be present during the patient's interview and examination and may answer questions for the patient. The health care professional should include the eldest family member present in the discussion. Individual responsibility for health actions and signing informed consent forms are reserved for those with expert knowledge; therefore the patient's signature may not *mean* that informed permission has been given.

Dominance Patterns: Male-dominated.

Eye Contact Practices: Observing the eyes at close range (approximately 2 feet) during conversation permits evaluation. The pupil of the eye dilates with interest or contracts with dislike.

Touch Practices: Touch is an important part of communication. It is limited to members of the same sex.

Perceptions of Time: Time is oriented to the present because planning ahead contains the potential for defying God's will.

Pain Reactions: Pain relief is expected to be immediate and may be requested persistently. Therapies requiring exertion are incompatible with belief in energy conservation for recovery. Pain is expressed privately or in the company of close relatives or friends. The exception is during labor and delivery.

Birth Rites: Newborns are swaddled and dressed in a shirt called a jalabiya that is made by relatives. The grandmother stays close to the mother during the mother's hospital stay. A celebration, sponsored by the grandparents, is held on the infant's seventh day.

Death Rites: Hope is valued; therefore confronting the patient with a grave diagnosis shatters hope and creates mistrust. The belief is that only God knows the true prognosis, and no one must speak of death. Health care professionals may be asked to shield the patient with a terminal illness from the truth. At death, a Muslim should help the patient recite the Declaration of the Faith:

"There is no God but God, and Muhammed is his Messenger." Expressive, vocal wailing is acceptable. The family may prefer to stay in the room with the body to talk to the deceased and to reflect on the person's accomplishments. More time is needed with the death of a child to reminisce on what the child might have accomplished. Touching the body is part of the final farewell. Family members wash the body according to Islamic tradition. Muslim belief forbids organ donation or transplants. Muslim physicians may recommend transfusions to save lives. Autopsy is uncommon because the deceased must be buried intact. Cremation is not permitted. For Muslim burial the body is wrapped in special pieces of cloth and buried without a coffin in the ground.

Food Practices and Intolerances: The evening meal is taken at approximately 10 PM. Pork, carrion, and blood are forbidden. Food tends to be spicy. Ramadan fasting is practiced between sunrise and sunset, with exemptions for the sick and for children.

National Childhood Immunizations: OPV-1 at 2 months; OPV-2 at 4 months; OPV-3 at 6 months; OPV booster between 15 and 24 months; BCG at birth to 3 months; DPT-1 at 2 months; DPT-2 at 4 months; DPT-3 at 6 months; DPT boosters between 18 and 24 months; DT-1 at 6 years or at entry into school; DT-2 at 10 years; measles at 9 months.

Other Characteristics: Female circumcision is viewed as the ultimate proof of virginity. The practice is still performed in more traditional or remote areas when a girl is 7 or 8 years old. Menarche may occur later than 15 years of age. Verbal consent is equal to written consent; pressing for written consent suggests mistrust of a verbal contract and is an insult to an individual's honor. Hope, optimism, and the positive advantages of treatment should be stressed when discussing outcomes. Some women retain their surname after marriage.

BIBLIOGRAPHY

Brown Y: Female circumcision, *Can Nurse* Apr:19, 1989.
Davis CF: Culturally responsive nursing management in an international health care setting, *Nurs Admin Q* 16(2):36, 1992.

Gadalla S, McCarthy J, Campbell O: How the number of living sons influences contraceptive use in Menoufia Governorate, Egypt, *Stud Fam Plann* 16(3):164, 1985.

Galanti GA: *Caring for patients from different cultures,* Philadelphia, 1991, University of Pennsylvania Press.

Gary R: Nurse development program, *Nurs Adm Q* 16(2):25, 1992.

Govaerts K, Patino E: Attachment behavior of the Egyptian mother, *Int J Nurs Stud* 18:53, 1981.

Green J: Death with dignity: Islam, *Nurs Times* 85(5):56, 1989.

Hall ET: Learning the Arabs' silent language, *Psychol Today* Aug:45, 1979.

Hathout MM: Comment on ethical crises and cultural differences, *West J Med* 139(3):380, 1983.

Lally MM: Last rites and funeral customs of minority groups, *Midwife Health Visit Comm Nurse* 14(7):224, 1978.

Meleis AI: The Arab American in the health care system, *Am J Nurs* June:1180, 1981.

Meleis AI, Jonsen AR: Medicine in perspective: ethical crises and cultural differences, *West J Med* 138(6):889, 1983.

Meleis AI, LaFever CW: The Arab American psychiatric care, *Perspec Psychiatr Care* 22(2):72, 1984.

Meleis AI, Sorrell L: Arab American women and their birth experiences, *MCN* 6:171, 1981.

Overfield T: *Biologic variation in health and illness,* Menlo Park, Calif, 1985, Addison-Wesley.

Reizian A, Meleis AI: Arab-Americans' perceptions of and responses to pain, *Crit Care Nurse* 6(6):30, 1986.

Ross HM: Societal/cultural views regarding death and dying, *Top Clin Nurs* 1(1):1, 1981.

Segall ME: Return to Aswan: picking up the threads, *Int Nurs Rev* 32(3):84, 1985.

Segall ME: Return to Aswan: planning the course, *Int Nurs Rev* 32(4):109, 1985.

◆ EL SALVADOR

MAP PAGE (256)

Location: This smallest of the Central American countries is situated on the Pacific coast, and much of the land is a fertile volcanic plateau.

Major Languages	Ethnic Groups		Major Religions	
Spanish	Mestizo	89%	Catholic	97%
Nahua	Native		Other	3%
	American	10%		
	White	1%		

Predominant Sick Care Practices: Biomedical.

Health Care Beliefs: Fresh air, sleep, and good nutrition are important health practices.

Ethnic/Race Specific or Endemic Diseases: ENDEMIC: Chloroquine-sensitive malaria. No risk in urban areas.

Food Practices and Intolerances: Some believe that being thin is unhealthy and weight control is not equated with good nutrition.

National Childhood Immunizations: DPT-1 at 3 months; DPT-2 at 6 months; DPT-3 at 9 months; DPT boosters at 1½ years and 5 years; OPV-1 at 2 months; OPV-2 at 4 months; OPV-3 at 6 months; two OPV boosters are administered (times not stated); measles at 9 months; BCG at birth and 7 years.

BIBLIOGRAPHY

Boyle JS: Constructs of health promotion and wellness in a Salvadoran population, *Pub Health Nurs* 6(3):129, 1989.

Boyle JS, Andrews MM: *Transcultural concepts in nursing care,* Glenview, Ill, 1989, Scott, Foresman/Little, Brown College Division.

Liveoak V: A Texas RN in El Salvador, *Texas Nurse* 63(6):12, 1989.

Tigerman NS: Health beliefs, knowledge and health seeking behaviors of recently immigrated Central American mothers in Los Angeles (California). Doctoral dissertation, Los Angeles, 1988, University of California.

Umanzor S: Nightmare in El Salvador: a nursing student's story, *J Christ Nurs* 3(2):10, 1986.

Zadel J: Nurse returns after three years in El Salvador, *Chart* 82(10):1, 1985.

◆ EQUATORIAL GUINEA

MAP PAGE (261)

Location: Equatorial Guinea, formerly Spanish Guinea, is located on the western coast of Africa. This nation includes several islands in the Gulf of Guinea.

Major Languages	Ethnic Groups		Major Religions	
Spanish	Fang	60%	Catholic	60%
Pidgin English	Bubi	30%	Indigenous	
Fang	Other	10%	and Other	40%

Ethnic/Race Specific or Endemic Diseases: ENDEMIC: Yellow fever; chloroquine-resistant malaria. RISK: Schistosomiasis.

National Childhood Immunizations: BCG at birth; DPT-1 at 3 months; DPT-2 at 4 months; DPT-3 at 5 months; measles at 9 months; OPV-1 at 3 months; OPV-2 at 4 months; OPV-3 at 5 months.

BIBLIOGRAPHY

No data located.

◆ ETHIOPIA

MAP PAGE (260)

Location: Black Africa's oldest state is located in east central Africa and borders the Red Sea on the north. Subsistence farming is severely affected by drought.

Major Languages	Ethnic Groups		Major Religions	
Amharic	Oromo	40%	Muslim	45%
Tigrinya	Amhara and		Ethiopian	
Orominga	Tigrean	32%	Orthodox	35%
Arabic	Sidamo	9%	Animist	
English	Shankella	6%	and Other	20%
	Somali			
	and Other	13%		

Predominant Sick Care Practices: Magico-religious. Some local practices may include wearing amulets (protection against disease) and bloodletting to treat malaria.

Ethnic/Race Specific or Endemic Diseases: ENDEMIC: Chloroquine-resistant malaria, with the exception of Addis Ababa; yellow fever. RISK: Schistosomiasis; pneumonia; postmeasles complications; malnutrition; anemia; intestinal parasites; diarrhea; eye infections; vitamins A and B deficiencies, including night blindness. ACTIVE: Leprosy.

Families' Role in Hospital Care: Families may move into the hospital and help with the patient's physical care.

Touch Practices: Spitting on a child while remarking on his or her good looks prevents inadvertently casting the evil eye.

Birth Rites: During the first hours after birth, the mother may turn away from the infant—a symbolic rejection for the pain the infant caused during birth. The mother remains confined for 14 to 40 days.

Death Rites: Muslim belief forbids organ donation or transplants. Muslim physicians may recommend transfusions to save lives. Autopsy is uncommon because the deceased must be buried intact. Cremation is not permitted. For Muslim burial the body is wrapped in special pieces of cloth and buried without a coffin in the ground. Loud wailing is a normal grief reaction.

Food Practices and Intolerances: Some do not eat chicken, considering it dirty.

Infant Feeding Practices: Sugar and water are given instead of colostrum, which is believed to be bad for the newborn. Food and fluids may be withheld from children to treat diarrhea.

Child Rearing Practices: Children who are ill may be kept lying in one place until they get better.

National Childhood Immunizations: BCG at birth; DPT-1 at 6 weeks; DPT-2 at 10 weeks; DPT-3 at 14 weeks;

measles at 9 months; OPV-1 at 6 weeks; OPV-2 at 10 weeks; OPV-3 at 14 weeks.

BIBLIOGRAPHY

Galanti GA: *Caring for patients from different cultures,* Philadelphia, 1991, University of Pennsylvania Press.

Hartz J: Children in exile, NBC-TV, March 8, 1992.

Kingham T: War babies, *Nurs Times* 86(3):28, 1990.

Ross HM: Societal/cultural views regarding death and dying, *Top Clin Nurs* 1(1):1, 1981.

Stuhr D: Destination Ethiopia, *J Christ Nurs* 3(4):28, 1986.

Trites P: Ethiopian experience, *Can Nurse* Nov:13, 1985.

Wallace C: A day in clinic and hospital, *Can Nurse* Oct:36, 1988.

◆ FIJI

MAP PAGE (255)

Location: More than 500 islands in the southern Pacific (about 2000 miles east of Australia) make up Fiji.

Major Languages	Ethnic Groups		Major Religions	
English	East Indian	49%	Christian	52%
Fijian	Fijian	46%	Hindu	42%
Hindustani	European and		Muslim	4%
	Other	5%	Other	2%

Ethnic/Race Specific or Endemic Diseases: RISK: Dengue.

National Childhood Immunizations: BCG at birth, 5 years, and 12 years; measles at 9 months; rubella at 12 years for girls; DPT at 2 months, 3 months, and 4 months; DT between 5 and 6 years; polio at 3 months, between 5 and 6 months, and at 9 months, with a booster at school entry.

Other Characteristics: It is considered impolite to raise the arms while talking to someone. Talking with the arms crossed over the chest is a sign of respect.

BIBLIOGRAPHY

Andy TC: The utilisation of a primary health care centre on an isolated island: Cicia, Fiji, *Cent Afr J Med* 36(10):246, 1990.

◆ FINLAND

MAP PAGE (258)

Location: Finland stretches about 700 miles (1126 km) north and south from the Arctic Circle to the Gulf of Finland, with Russia along its eastern border. It is the second most northern country in the world, with long, cold winters.

Major Languages	Ethnic Groups		Major Religions	
Finnish	Finnish	93%	Lutheran	97%
Swedish	Swedish and		Greek	
Lapp	Other	7%	Orthodox	1%
Russian			Other	2%

Predominant Sick Care Practices: Biomedical.

Health Care Beliefs: Active involvement; health promotion is important.

Ethnic/Race Specific or Endemic Diseases: RISK: Congenital nephrosis; generalized amyloidosis syndrome; polycystic liver disease; cardiovascular diseases; cancer.

Dominance Patterns: Males may have slight dominance in some families; however, in making health care decisions for children, husband and wife share responsibility.

Eye Contact Practices: Direct eye contact, but it is held intermittently.

Touch Practices: Most touch infrequently; however, young couples often touch more frequently.

Time Perceptions: People are usually punctual and may be irritated by tardiness.

Pain Reactions: People are willing to communicate pain; however, they are not expressive.

Birth Rites: A midwife-assisted hospital birth predominates, with one of the lowest infant mortality rates in the industrialized world.

Death Rites: Relatives desire to be at the bedside of the dying person to pay final respects. Funeral directors provide all postmortem care. Burial in the ground is the common practice and is held several days after the death is announced in newspapers.

Food Practices and Intolerances: Coffee, sandwiches of meat and cheese, and porridge are common for breakfast. Lunch is the main meal. A small meal of coffee and sandwiches is taken after work. Reindeer meat is popular.

Infant Feeding Practices: Breastfeeding is common.

Child Rearing Practices: Free dental care is provided until age 18 and free health care, from birth to school age. Compulsory military service begins for boys at age 19. Two full meals are offered to children at school.

National Childhood Immunizations: BCG at birth (in the hospital) or at 3 months; DPT-1 at 3 months; DPT-2 at 4 months; DPT-3 at 5 months; DPT booster between 20 and 24 months; Td between 11 and 13 years; MMR between 14 and 18 months and at 6 years; injectable polio at 6 months, 12 months, 6 years, 11 years, and between 16 and 18 years.

Other Characteristics: Carrying on a conversation with hands in the pockets is impolite. The term *health center* means an organization of services rather than a building.

BIBLIOGRAPHY

Boyle JS, Andrews MM: *Transcultural concepts in nursing care,* Glenview, Ill, 1989, Scott, Foresman/Little, Brown College Division.

Carr C: A four-week observation of maternity care in Finland, *J Obstet Gynecol Neonat Nurs* 18(2):100, 1989.

Forni PR: Health care delivery in Sweden and Finland: a challenge to the American system, *J Prof Nurs* 2(4):234, 1986.

Geissler EM: Personal observations, August 5-11, 1992.

Lammi UK et al: Functional capacity and associated factors in elderly Finnish men, *Scand J Soc Med* 17(1):67, 1989.

Lindquist GJ: Primary health care in four countries, *J Prof Nurs* 2(4):203, 1986.

Pietinen P et al: Nutrition as a component in community control of cardiovascular disease, *Am J Clin Nutr* 49(5 Suppl):1017, 1989.

Rautava P et al: The Finnish family competence study: childbearing attitudes in pregnant nulliparae, *Acta Paedopsychiatr* 55(1):3, 1992.

Teperi J, Rimpela M: Menstrual pain, health and behaviour in girls, *Soc Sci Med* 29(2):163, 1989.

Valkama E: Personal communication, August 5, 1992.

Virgin C, Jacobsen U: More female warmth and less high technology. Paper presented at the Fifth International Council on Women's Health Issues, Copenhagen, 1992.

◆ FRANCE

MAP PAGE (258)

Location: The second largest European nation, France is mountainous in the extreme east and consists of river basins and a plateau throughout the rest of the nation.

Major Languages	Ethnic Groups		Major Religions	
French	French	97%	Catholic	90%
Alsatian	Other	3%	Protestant	2%
Breton			Jewish	1%
Corsican			Muslim	1%
Basque			Unaffiliated and Other	6%

Health Care Beliefs: Eating proper food, wearing proper clothing, resting and taking cod liver oil daily are believed to promote health.

Health Team Relationships: When meeting people, protocol is observed and behavior is polite. Titles and status are important. First names should not be used. Engaging in general conversation to establish social contact is acceptable. Often, details are not included in communications, and hidden meanings may not be verbalized. Giving logical, sequential reasons for actions is important to ensure the patient's compliance. Rules and regulations may be circumvented to reach a goal.

Eye Contact Practices: Direct eye contact is maintained. The face is expressive, as are gestures.

Touch Practices: The French touch frequently. The southern French prefer closeness during conversation. Handshaking and a kiss on each cheek when greeting or leaving is common.

Time Perceptions: The present is viewed in the context of French history. Strict adherence to schedules is not routinely expected; changing plans at the last minute is acceptable.

Death Rites: Chrysanthemums are used exclusively for funerals.

Food Practices and Intolerances: The main meal is usually at noon if that time is compatible with work schedules. A loaf of bread is torn rather than sliced.

National Childhood Immunizations: BCG at one month, before 6th birthday, between 11 and 13 years, and between 16 and 21 years for negative reactors; DPT-1 at 2 months; DPT-2 at 3 months; DPT-3 at 4 months; DPT booster between 15 and 18 months; DT between 5 and 6 years and 16 and 21 years; injectable polio at 2 months, 3 months, 4 months, between 15 and 18 months, between 11 and 13 years, and between 16 and 21 years; MMR at 12 months, between 5 and 6 years; mumps for unvaccinated boys between 11 and 13 years; rubella for all girls between 11 and 13 years.

Other Characteristics: Carrying on a conversation with the hands in the pockets is not received well. Only written formal agreements are considered binding.

BIBLIOGRAPHY

Giger JN, Davidhizar RE: *Transcultural Nursing,* St Louis, 1991, Mosby.
Hall ET, Hall MR: *Understanding cultural differences: Germans, French and Americans,* Yarmouth, Me, 1990, Intercultural Press.
Prosser MH: *The cultural dialogue,* Washington, DC, 1985, SIETAR.
Samovar LA, Porter RE: *Intercultural communication: a reader,* Belmont, Calif, 1985, Wadsworth.
Spector RE: *Cultural diversity in health and illness,* ed 3, Norwalk, Conn, 1991, Appleton & Lange.

Storti C: *The art of crossing cultures,* Yarmouth, Me, 1990, Intercultural Press.

◆ FRENCH GUIANA

MAP PAGE (258)

Location: This overseas department of France is located on the northeast coast of South America. Timber rain forests cover most of this largely undeveloped land, and the climate is tropical. Most of the population live along the Atlantic coast and are descendants of African slaves.

Major Language	Ethnic Groups		Major Religions	
French	Black/		Catholic	80%
	Mulatto	66%	Indigenous and	
	White	12%	Other	20%
	Asian	12%		
	Other	10%		

Ethnic/Race Specific or Endemic Diseases: ENDEMIC: Chloroquine-resistant malaria; yellow fever. AIDS case rate is 46.6/100,000 people.

BIBLIOGRAPHY

Adler MW, editor: Statistics from the World Health Organization and the Centers for Disease Control, *AIDS* 6(10):1229, 1992.

◆ GABON

MAP PAGE (261)

Location: This West African nation sits astride the equator along the Atlantic seaboard. Most of the country is covered by dense tropical forest.

Major Languages	Ethnic Groups		Major Religions	
French	Fang	25%	Christian	60%
Fang	Bapounou	10%	Muslim	1%
Myene	Other	65%	Indigenous	
			and Other	39%

Ethnic/Race Specific or Endemic Diseases: ENDEMIC: Chloroquine-resistant malaria; yellow fever. RISK: Schistosomiasis.

National Childhood Immunizations: BCG at birth; DPT-1 at 6 weeks; DPT-2 at 10 weeks; DPT-3 at 14 weeks; measles at 9 months; OPV at birth; OPV-1 at 6 weeks; OPV-2 at 10 weeks; OPV-3 at 14 weeks.

BIBLIOGRAPHY

No data located.

◆ GAMBIA

MAP PAGE (260)

Location: Referred to as The Gambia, this smallest country of Africa is located on the Atlantic coast. The country is primarily savanna and is bisected by the wide Gambia River. Most major health care facilities are located on the south side of the river. Many people live at a subsistence level in bush villages.

Major Languages	Ethnic Groups		Major Religions	
English	Mandinka	42%	Muslim	90%
Mandinka	Fula	18%	Christian	9%
Wolof	Wolof	16%	Other	1%
Fula	Jola	10%		
Other	Serahuli			
	and Other	14%		

Predominant Sick Care Practices: Biomedical; magico-religious; traditional.

Health Care Beliefs: Health promotion is important. The country's primary health care plan is considered an excellent model by other developing countries.

Ethnic/Race Specific or Endemic Diseases: ACTIVE: Yellow fever. ENDEMIC: Chloroquine-resistant malaria (including urban areas). RISK: Schistosomiasis; tuberculosis; most young children are pneumococcus carriers. Infant, child, and maternal mortality rates are high. Hemoglobin levels below 10 g are common.

Birth Rites: Both squatting and supine positions are used for birthing. Some believe that the father must provide the razor blade used to cut the umbilical cord. A special naming celebration with drums and dancing is held on the eighth day. A witch doctor *(Maribou)* provides small leather pouches containing holy verses to be secured on a string and worn around the infant's neck for protection.

Death Rites: Muslim belief forbids organ donation or transplants. Muslim physicians may recommend transfusions to save lives. Autopsy is uncommon because the deceased must be buried intact. Cremation is not permitted. For Muslim burial the body is wrapped in special pieces of cloth and buried without a coffin in the ground.

Infant Feeding Practices: The newborn is given only warm water the first day. Breastfeeding is started the second day.

Child Rearing Practices: Family planning may not be acceptable.

National Childhood Immunizations: BCG at birth; DPT-1 at 2 months; DPT-2 at 3 months; DPT-3 at 4 months; DPT booster at 16 months; measles and yellow fever at 9 months; OPV at birth; OPV-1 at 2 months; OPV-2 at 3 months; OPV-3 at 4 months; OPV-4 at 9 months.

BIBLIOGRAPHY

Campbell H, Byass P, Greenwood BM: Acute lower respiratory infections in Gambian children: maternal perception of illness, *Ann Trop Paediatr* 10(1):45, 1990.

Daly C, Pollard AJ: Traditional birth attendants in The Gambia, *Midwives Chron* 103(1227):104, 1990.

Gudmundsen AM: Building an infrastructure for international health promotion and disease prevention: the Peace Corps fellows program, *J Prof Nurs* 5(4):172, 1989.

Ho E: Midwifery training and practice in The Gambia, *Midwives Chron* 100(1191):109, 1987.

Ross HM: Societal/cultural views regarding death and dying, *Top Clin Nurs* 1(1):1, 1981.

Slack P: Built on tradition, *Nurs Times* 84(47):40, 1988.

◆ GERMANY

MAP PAGE (258)

Location: Following World War II, Germany was divided, with East Germany (German Democratic Republic) going to the Soviet Union and West Germany (Federal Republic of Germany) occupied by the United States. Reunification took place on October 3, 1990.

Major Languages	Ethnic Groups		Major Religions	
[Former East Germany]	German	99%	Protestant	47%
	Slavic		Catholic	7%
German	and Other	1%	Unaffiliated	
			and Other	46%
[Former West Germany]				
German	German	93%	Protestant	49%
	Turkish	2%	Catholic	45%
	Italian		Other	6%
	and Other	5%		

Predominant Sick Care Practices: Biomedical; magico-religious. Younger people tend to oppose technical medicine and consult, instead, herbalists. The evil eye and God are thought by some to cause illness.

Health Care Beliefs: Active involvement; passive role; health promotion is important. Older people tend to take a passive health care role. Former East Germans may demonstrate less responsibility for their health promotion and care.

Ethnic/Race Specific or Endemic Diseases: RISK: Bordetella pertussis (whooping cough) in parts of West Germany.

Health Team Relationships: Introductory social conversation is not encouraged; instead getting to the immediate issue is common. Patients often address the health professional by title rather than name. Patients may not ask questions of a health professional because this would be a challenge to that authority. Information may not be shared freely.

Dominance Patterns: Male and female share responsibility in decision-making; children can be involved in decision-making. Many married women do not work outside the home.

Eye Contact Practices: Sustained direct eye contact indicates that the person listens, trusts, is somewhat aggressive, or, in some situations, is sexually interested. Looking inside a room is considered the same as entering the room; therefore doors are often kept closed.

Touch Practices: Touch is infrequent. A handshake is common at the beginning and end of an interaction.

Time Perceptions: Punctuality in all situations is maintained. People are oriented to the present and to the near future. A strong consciousness of history is exhibited, particularly in the older generation. Business people end work promptly at 5 PM.

Pain Reactions: Strong, stoic behavior is exhibited. If feeling the pain is perceived as part of the healing process, it may be tolerated; otherwise, relief of pain is desired.

Birth Rites: Most deliveries occur in hospitals; the father may choose to be present during birth. Courses for natural childbirth, prenatal care, and postnatal care are popular.

Death Rites: Crying in private is expected. Cremation is becoming popular. A possible delay of 3 days to a week before burial may occur because of the bureaucratic processing of paperwork. German society tends to put the elderly in long-term care facilities.

Food Practices and Intolerances: Traditionally lunch is the preferred main meal; however, for working families, it is dinner. Potatoes, vegetables, bread, and thick soups are common. Champagne, beer, soft drinks, and meat are popular. Rolls are served only at breakfast, with cheese or ham. Hot coffee or tea is the morning beverage. Mealtime is the time to enjoy discussing political or intellectual issues.

Infant Feeding Practices: Breastfeeding is common, with bottle feeding introduced at 6 months to 1 year.

Child Rearing Practices: Mild discipline using reasoning to influence behavior is common.

National Childhood Immunizations: DPT or DT at 3 months, 4 months, and 15 months; DT and adult tetanus between 6 and 8 years; OPV at 3 months, 4½ months, and 10 years; MMR at 15 months; rubella for girls between 10 and 15 years; Td between 6 and 8 years and 10 and 15 years.

Other Characteristics: Privacy, formality, and social distance are highly valued. With reunification, respect for the former East German sector is important. The thumbs up gesture may mean the number one.

BIBLIOGRAPHY

Bueche MN: Maternal-infant health care: a comparison between the United States and West Germany, *Nurs Forum* 25(4):25, 1990.

Condon JC, Yousef F: *An introduction to intercultural communication,* New York, 1975, Macmillan.

Dopson L: Health care in Germany, *Nurs Times* 84(17):33, 1988.

Finger H et al: The epidemiological situation of pertussis in the Federal Republic of Germany, *Dev Biol Stand* 73:343, 1991.

Galanti GA: *Caring for patients from different cultures,* Philadelphia, 1991, University of Pennsylvania Press.

Giger JN, Davidhizar RE: *Transcultural nursing,* St Louis, 1991, Mosby.

Goldberg RT: Comparison of the German and American systems of rehabilitation, *J Rehabil* 55(1):59, 1989.

Hall ET, Hall MR: *Understanding cultural differences: Germans, French and Americans,* Yarmouth, Me, 1990, Intercultural Press.

Language Research Center: *German-speaking people of Europe,* Provo, Utah, 1976, Brigham Young University.

Luegenbiehl DL: The birth system in Germany, *JOGNN* 14(1):45, 1985.

Prosser MH: *The cultural dialogue,* Washington, DC, 1985, SIETAR.

Rieke HJ: Contributor.

Samovar LA, Porter RE: *Intercultural communication: a reader,* Belmont, Calif, 1985, Wadsworth.

Spector RE: *Cultural diversity in health and illness,* ed 3, Norwalk, Conn, 1991, Appleton & Lange.

Stewart EC, Bennett MJ: *American cultural patterns: a cross-cultural perspective,* rev ed, Yarmouth, Me, 1991, Intercultural Press.

Tinsley RL Jr, Woloshin DJ: Approaching German culture: a tentative analysis, Reprint from *Die Unterrichtspraxis* 3(1):125, 1974.

Whetstone WR: Perceptions of self-care in East Germany: a cross-cultural empirical investigation, *J Adv Nurs* 12:167, 1987.

◆ GHANA

MAP PAGE (260)

Location: Ghana was formerly the Gold Coast. Its southern border lies along the Gulf of Guinea in West Africa. The majority of people are black Africans with many different languages and with a diverse ethnicity.

Major Languages	Ethnic Groups		Major Religions	
English	Akan	44%	Indigenous	
Akan	Moshi-		Beliefs	38%
Moshi-	Dagomba	16%	Muslim	30%
Dagomba	Ewe	13%	Christian	24%
Ewe	Ga	8%	Other	8%
Ga	Other	19%		

Ethnic/Race Specific or Endemic Diseases: ACTIVE: Cholera, yellow fever. ENDEMIC: Chloroquine-resistant malaria; schistosomiasis; Guinea worm disease.

Health Team Relationships: Mass media, churches, and religious organizations teach health education as information flows routinely from the Ministry of Health. A town crier, also known as a "gong man," passes health information along in rural areas.

Families' Role in Hospital Care: Families may wash and cook for the patient. Some believe that hospitals are places to go to die.

Dominance Patterns: It is a polygamous society; however, men do not socialize with their wives. Some tribes are matrilineal.

Eye Contact Practices: Staring is taboo; however, direct eye contact is used in conversations.

Touch Practices: Men and women touch frequently in this culture.

Time Perceptions: Punctuality is not important. Continuing a social interaction is more important than being punctual at another event.

Birth Rites: Once they are assured the baby is alive and well, mothers may not look at their infants for a while.

Food Practices and Intolerances: The main meal of the three is in the evening. The staple food is boiled root crops mixed together. Fruit is eaten, often as a dessert. The right hand is used to eat because the left hand is used to clean oneself after elimination.

Infant Feeding Practices: Breastfeeding is almost universal.

National Childhood Immunizations: BCG at birth; DPT-1 at 6 weeks; DPT-2 at 10 weeks; DPT-3 at 14 weeks; measles at 9 months; OPV at birth; OPV-1 at 6 weeks; OPV-2 at 10 weeks; OPV-3 at 14 weeks.

BIBLIOGRAPHY

Bosompra K: Dissemination of health information among rural dwellers in Africa: a Ghanaian experience, *Soc Sci Med* 29(9):1133, 1989.

Bowditch, Susan: Personal communication, July 24, 1991, Portland, Oregon.

McGinn T et al: Private midwives: a new approach to family planning service delivery in Ghana, *Midwifery* 6(3):117, 1990.

Osae-Addae M: Pain management of cancer in Ghana, *Cancer Nurs* 14(4):218, 1990.

Winsor C: A volunteer in Ghana, *Nurs Times* May 18:8, 1983.

◆ GREECE

MAP PAGE (258)

Location: Situated on the Mediterranean Sea, Greece is the southernmost country on the Balkan Peninsula in southern Europe.

Major Languages	Ethnic Groups		Major Religions	
Greek	Greek	98%	Greek Orthodox	98%
English	Turkish	1%	Muslim	1%
French	Other	1%	Other	1%

Predominant Sick Care Practices: Biomedical; magico-religious.

Health Care Beliefs: The evil eye is usually cast by witches. Protective blue beads or stone charms are worn. Garlic or onions may be hung in the traditional home or worn on the body to prevent illness.

Ethnic/Race Specific or Endemic Diseases: RISK: Mediterranean-type G6PD deficiency; β-thalassemia; familial Mediterranean fever.

Health Team Relationships: Nursing is not a valued profession.

Dominance Patterns: Love of family and respect for elders are strong values.

Eye Contact Practices: Staring in public is acceptable.

Pain Reactions: Passive reactions to pain is practiced.

Death Rites: The dying may be physically isolated, and truth of a terminal diagnosis withheld. Death at home is important. Folk culture incorporates a dread of death. Death rites serve to maintain a social relationship with the deceased. Children are not excluded from the rituals. Traditionally, a relative or elderly woman washes the body with water or wine. Rituals are not concluded until the body has been exhumed 5 years after death and the bones have been placed in an urn or a vault. For the rest of her life a widow wears dark mourning clothes. The widow's social support systems may span several generations, providing food, hospitality, and companionship.

Food Practices and Intolerances: The main meal of the day is at noon.

Child Rearing Practices: Parents may be overprotective of daughters. Children depend heavily on the family.

National Childhood Immunizations: DPT at 2 months, 4 months, 6 months, 18 months, and between 4 and 6 years; TOPV at 2 months, 4 months, 6 months, 18 months, and between 4 and 6 years; MMR or measles vaccine at 15 months; BCG between 6 and 14 years; tetanus toxoid between 12 and 14 years.

Other Characteristics: The head motions for "yes" and "no" are opposite those used in the United States. Because a man's body hair is linked to manhood, shaving body hair for treatments may be resisted or refused.

BIBLIOGRAPHY

Boyle JS, Andrews MM: *Transcultural concepts in nursing care,* Glenview, Ill, 1989, Scott, Foresman/Little, Brown College Division.

Dracopoulou S, Doxiadis S: Care of the dying in Greece: lament for the dead, denial for the dying, *Hastings Center Rep* Aug:15, 1988.

Eisenbruch M: Cross-cultural aspects of bereavement, Part 2, ethnic and cultural variations in the development of bereavement practices, *Cult Med Psychiatry* 8(4):315, 1984.

Ierodiakonou CS: Adolescents' mental health and the Greek family: preventive aspects, *J Adolesc* 11(1):11, 1988.

Irujo S: *An introduction to intercultural differences and similarities in nonverbal communication.* In Wurzel JS: *Toward multiculturalism,* Yarmouth, Me, 1988, Intercultural Press.

Lofvander M, Papastavrou D: Clinical factors, psycho-social stressors and sick-leave patterns in a group of Swedish and Greek patients, *Scand J Soc Med* 18(2):133, 1990.

Parker G, Lipscombe P: Parental characteristics of Jews and Greeks in Australia, *Aust NZ J Psychiatry* 13(3):225, 1979.

Rosenbaum JN: Cultural care of older Greek Canadian widows within Leininger's theory of culture care, *J Transcult Nurs* 2(1):37, 1990.

Rosenbaum JN: The health meanings and practices of older Greek-Canadian widows, *J Adv Nurs* 16(11):1320, 1991.

Solomon J: Critical care nursing, *Focus Crit Care* 13(3):10, 1986.

Spector RE: *Cultural diversity in health and illness,* ed 3, Norwalk, Conn, 1991, Appleton & Lange.

Tripp-Reimer T: Retention of folk-healing practice (Matiasma) among four generations of urban Greek immigrants, *Nurs Res* 32(2):97, 1983.

◆ GRENADA

MAP PAGE (257)

Location: Located 100 miles from the South American coast, Grenada is the southernmost of the Caribbean Windward Islands.

Major Languages	Ethnic Groups		Major Religions	
English	African	99%	Catholic	68%
French Patois	Other	1%	Anglican	23%
			Other	9%

BIBLIOGRAPHY

DeVooght J, Walker K: Community mental health care in Grenada, *Int Nurs Rev* 36(1):22, 1989.

Walker K, DeVooght J: Invasion — new psychiatric facility: Grenada, *J Psychosoc Nurs Ment Health Serv* 27(1):37, 1989.

◆ GUATEMALA

MAP PAGE (256)

Location: Bordered on the north, west, and east by Mexico, Guatemala is the northernmost of the Central American nations. The cool highlands contain the heaviest population. The lands bordering the Caribbean and Pacific are tropical.

Major Languages	Ethnic Groups		Major Religions	
Spanish	Ladino	56%	Catholic	88%
Indian	Native		Mayan	
Languages	American		and Other	12%
	and Other	44%		

Predominant Sick Care Practices: Traditional herbs are incorporated into some health care. The *nervo forza* is a popular liquid vitamin taken to promote health.

Health Care Beliefs: Acute sick care only. Measures to cure acute problems are valued and are linked to preventive measures by some health care practitioners.

Ethnic/Race Specific or Endemic Diseases: ENDEMIC: Chloroquine-sensitive malaria; filaria. RISK: Malnutrition; diarrhea; lower respiratory tract infections; measles in young children.

Health Team Relationships: Attempts to institute primary health care are strongly opposed.

Time Perceptions: Punctuality is not valued.

National Childhood Immunizations: DPT-1 at 3 months; DPT-2 at 6 months; DPT-3 at 9 months; OPV-1 at 3 months; OPV-2 at 6 months; OPV-3 at 9 months; measles at 9 months; BCG between birth and 5 years.

BIBLIOGRAPHY

Annel MV: Overview—experience and community participation count in Guatemala, *Pub Health Rev* 12(3-4):261, 1984.

Boyle JS: *Caring practices in a Guatemalan Colonia.* In Leininger MM: *Care: the essence of nursing and health,* Thorofare, NJ, 1984, SLACK.

Boyle JS: Ideology and illness experiences of women in Guatemala, *Health Care Women Int* 6(1-3):73, 1985.

Broach J, Newton N: Food and beverages in labor, Part 1, cross-cultural and historical practices, *Birth* 15(2):81, 1988.

Glittenberg J: Adapting health care to a cultural setting, *Am J Nurs* 74(12):2218, 1974.

Heggenhougen HK: Will primary health care efforts be allowed to succeed? *Soc Sci Med* 19(3):217, 1984.

Lechtig A et al: Nutrition, family planning, and health promotion: the Guatemalan program of primary health care, *Birth* 9(2):97, 1982.

Richards F et al: Knowledge, attitudes and perceptions (KAP) of onchocerciasis: a survey among residents in an endemic area in Guatemala, *Soc Sci Med* 32(11):1275, 1991.

Spector RE: *Cultural diversity in health and illness,* ed 3, Norwalk, Conn, 1991, Appleton & Lange.

Stewart EC, Bennett MJ: *American cultural patterns: a cross-cultural perspective,* rev ed, Yarmouth, Me, 1991, Intercultural Press.

◆ GUINEA

MAP PAGE (260)

Location: This West African nation is located on the Atlantic and consists of a coastal plain, a mountainous region, a savanna interior, and a forest in the Guinea Highlands.

Major Languages	Ethnic Groups		Major Religions	
French	Fulani	40%	Muslim	85%
African	Malinke	25%	Christian	10%
Languages	Sousou	10%	Indigenous	
	Other	25%	Beliefs	5%

Ethnic/Race Specific or Endemic Diseases: ACTIVE: Cholera; yellow fever. RISK: Chloroquine-resistant malaria; schistosomiasis.

Death Rites: Muslim belief forbids organ donation or transplants. Muslim physicians may recommend transfusions to save lives. Autopsy is uncommon because the deceased must be buried intact. Cremation is not permitted. For Muslim burial the body is wrapped in special pieces of cloth and buried without a coffin in the ground.

National Childhood Immunizations: BCG at birth; DPT-1 at 6 weeks; DPT-2 at 10 weeks; DPT-3 at 14 weeks; DPT booster at 6 years; measles at 9 months; OPV at birth; OPV-1 at 6 weeks; OPV-2 at 10 weeks; OPV-3 at 14 weeks.

BIBLIOGRAPHY

Ross HM: Societal/cultural views regarding death and dying, *Top Clin Nurs* 1(1):1, 1981.

◆ GUINEA-BISSAU

MAP PAGE (260)

Location: Formerly Portuguese Guiana, Guinea-Bissau is located on the Atlantic coast of West Africa. Most of the country consists of rain forests, swamps, and mangrove-covered wetlands.

Major Languages	Ethnic Groups		Major Religions	
Portuguese	Balanta	30%	Indigenous	
Crioulo	Fulani	20%	Beliefs	65%
Other	Manjaca	14%	Muslim	30%
	Mandinga	13%	Christian	5%
	Papel			
	and Other	23%		

Ethnic/Race Specific or Endemic Diseases: ENDEMIC: Chloroquine-resistant malaria; yellow fever. RISK: Schistosomiasis.

National Childhood Immunizations: BCG at birth; measles at 9 months; yellow fever at 12½ months; DPT-1 at 3 months; DPT-2 at 4 months; DPT-3 at 5 months; OPV-1 at 3 months; OPV-2 at 4 months; OPV-3 at 5 months.

BIBLIOGRAPHY

No data located.

◆ GUYANA

MAP PAGE (258)

Location: Formerly British Guiana, the country is located on the northern coast of South America. Ninety percent of the population lives in the low coastal areas. Highlands are in the south, and an extensive network of rivers runs from north to south.

Major Languages	Ethnic Groups		Major Religions	
English	East Indian	51%	Christian	57%
Indian	Black and		Hindu	33%
Languages	Mixed	43%	Muslim	9%
	Native		Other	1%
	American	4%		
	European and			
	Chinese	2%		

Ethnic/Race Specific or Endemic Diseases: ENDEMIC: Chloroquine-resistant malaria; yellow fever; filariasis.

BIBLIOGRAPHY

Nathan MB, Stroom V: Prevalence of *Wuchereria bancrofti* in Georgetown, Guyana, *Bull Pan Am Health Org* 24(3):301, 1990.

◆ HAITI

MAP PAGE (257)

Location: Located in the West Indies of the Caribbean, Haiti occupies the western one third of the island of Hispaniola, sharing it with the Dominican Republic. Much of the mountainous northern soil is denuded. Haiti is known as the poorest nation in the western hemisphere.

Major Languages	Ethnic Groups		Major Religions	
French	Black	95%	Catholic	80%
Creole	Mulatto and		Protestant	10%
	European	5%	Voodoo	10%

Officially listed above (Major Religions) as "Voodoo 10%," as many as 90% of the people believe, regardless of their religion.

Predominant Sick Care Practices: Biomedical; magico-religious. Western medical treatment is sought (including in rural areas) more often than traditional medicine is used. Belief in voodoo is important, as well as the belief in prayer and the healing power and protection of God against misfortune. Illnesses that are perceived to originate supernaturally or magically can be treated only with voodoo medicine. Ethnomedical beliefs about disease are based on maintenance of a hot/cold equilibrium within the body. Herbalists treat common disorders and specialize in the treatment of the evil eye *(maldyok)*.

Health Care Beliefs: Passive role; acute sick care only; health promotion is important. A traditional individual may evaluate his or her illness according to symptoms previously experienced by close relatives. Fatalistic attitudes may be present.

Ethnic/Race Specific or Endemic Diseases: ENDEMIC: Chloroquine-sensitive malaria. AIDS case rate is 9.7/ 100,000 people.

Health Team Relationships: The doctor is the primary authority, and nurses are subordinate in hospital settings. If nurses are the only health care professionals available, they are afforded more respect.

Families Role in Hospital Care: The family is required to stay with the patient and provide food and basic hygiene.

Dominance Patterns: The family is a mutual support system. Siblings remain close, even after marriage.

Eye Contact Practices: It is customary to hold eye contact with everyone except the poor.

Time Perceptions: Punctuality is not an important value. Hope for the future promotes a future-oriented view; however, the society is predominately oriented to the present.

Pain Reactions: A high tolerance for pain and discomfort exists.

Birth Rites: During pregnancy some believe that they must continue sexual intercourse to keep the birth canal lubricated or that they must avoid exposing themselves to cold air. Most babies are delivered at home with the mothers squatting or in a semiseated position. For believers in voodoo, the delivery is performed underneath a sheet because bright light during delivery is feared. Traditionalists may bury the placenta beneath the doorway at the birth site or burn it at a corner of the home. Postpartum confinement practices have decreased. Infants are not named until after the confinement month. If the infant dies during confinement, burial is done without ceremony. According to the hot/cold equilibrium theory, postpartum is the hottest state the body reaches, and mothers do not eat foods that are categorized as hot. Nutmeg, castor oil, or spider webs placed on the umbilical cord may contribute to neonatal tetanus. Belly bands are commonly used. Haiti has one of the highest infant mortality rates in the world.

Death Rites: Death is believed to be caused by natural or supernatural circumstances. Relatives and friends expend considerable effort to be present when death nears. The family does not express grief out loud until most of the deceased's possessions have been removed from the home; then wailing and crying begin. People who are knowledgeable in the customs wash, dress, and place the body in a coffin. A priest may be summoned to conduct the burial service. Burial usually takes place within 24 hours, with no embalming. A popular local belief alleges that witchdoctors use herbal substances to make people appear dead, bringing them back to life later to enslave them. Because of this popular story, doubts exist about whether a person is truly dead or merely appears dead. White clothing represents death. During grieving, some may assume the symptoms of the deceased's last illness.

Food Practices and Intolerances: The majority eat once a day. Water is taken only after the meal is finished.

Infant Feeding Practices: Colostrum is not considered good milk. Its use is encouraged as a purgative (instead of castor oil) to rid the infant's body of meconium. Some mothers stop breastfeeding if the infant develops diarrhea. Others believe that breast milk causes diarrhea or intestinal parasites. Breastfeeding is more common in rural areas and may be continued for 9 to 18 months. A plantain porridge supplement is given as early as 2 months.

Child Rearing Practices: It is customary to treat children in a harsh, strict manner, using corporal punishment. Children who ask questions or seek information from parents are thought to show disrespect for parental authority. When adults are speaking children are expected to remain quiet. Many children have multiple caretakers: relatives or friends. In cases of extreme poverty, children work after school to help support the family. Haitians are reluctant to discuss sex education or reproduction with those health care professionals who are not Haitian.

National Childhood Immunizations: DPT-1 at 6 weeks; DPT-2 at 4 months; DPT 3 at 5 months; DPT booster 1 year after DPT-3; OPV-1 at birth to 6 weeks; OPV-2 at 4 months; OPV-3 at 5 months; OPV booster 1 year after OPV-3; measles at 9 months; BCG at birth.

BIBLIOGRAPHY

Adler MW, editor: Statistics from the World Health Organization and the Centers for Disease Control, *AIDS* 6(10):1229, 1992.

Berggren WL, Ewbank DC, Berggren GG: Reduction of mortality in rural Haiti through a primary health care program, *N Engl J Med* 304:1324, 1981.

Berggren GG et al: Traditional midwives, tetanus immunization, and infant mortality in rural Haiti, *Trop Doc* Apr:79, 1983.

Boyle JS, Andrews MM: *Transcultural concepts in nursing care,* Glenview, Ill, 1989, Scott, Foresman/Little, Brown College Division.

Colman RM: *The Haitian immigrant community in Connecticut,* Storrs, 1985, University of Connecticut.

Coreil J: Allocation of family resources for health care in rural Haiti, *Medicine* 17(11):709, 1983.

DeSantis L: Bridging the gap: cultural diversity in nursing, Unpublished manuscript, 1990.

DeSantis L, Tappen RM: Preventive health practices of Haitian immigrants. Paper presented at the West Virginia Nurses Association research symposium, Sulphur Springs, W Va, 1990.

DeSantis L, Thomas JT: Parental attitudes toward adolescent sexuality: transcultural perspectives, *Nurs Pract* 12(8):43, 1987.

DeSantis L, Thomas JT: The immigrant Haitian mother: transcultural nursing perspective on preventive health care for children, *J Transcult Nurs* 2(1):2, 1990.

Eisenbruch M: Cross-cultural aspects of bereavement, Part 2, ethnic and cultural variations in the development of bereavement practices, *Cult Med Psychiatry* 8(4):315, 1984.

Gebrian B: Contributor.

King KW et al: Preventive and therapeutic benefits in relation to cost: performance over 10 years of mothercraft centers in Haiti, *J Clin Nutr* 31:679, 1978.

Kirkpatrick S, Cobb A: Health beliefs related to diarrhea in Haitian children: building transcultural nursing knowledge, *J Transcult Nurs* 1(2):2, 1990.

Li GR: *Funeral practices,* New York, World Relief, n.d.

Scalora S: *Haiti: flesh of politics, spirit of Vodun,* Storrs, 1991, University of Connecticut.

Smith-Campbell B: Haiti: an international nursing experience, *Kansas Nurse* Mar:4, 1988.

United Nations Children's Fund: *The status of the world's children, 1989,* Oxfordshire, United Kingdom, 1989, Oxford University Press.

◆ HONDURAS

MAP PAGE (256)

Location: Honduras is part of the north central section of Central America. Coastlines include the Caribbean Sea and the Pacific Ocean. Primarily mountainous, Honduras also has fertile plateaus, a river valley, and a narrow coastal plain.

Major Languages	Ethnic Groups		Major Religions	
Spanish	Mestizo	90%	Catholic	97%
Indian	Native		Protestant	
Languages	American	7%	and Other	3%
	Black	2%		
	White	1%		

Ethnic/Race Specific or Endemic Diseases: ENDEMIC: Chloroquine-sensitive malaria. **RISK:** Respiratory diseases. AIDS case rate is 11.4/100,000 people.

Dominance Patterns: Males dominate.

Infant Feeding Practices: The 1980s brought a marked increase in breastfeeding.

National Childhood Immunizations: DPT-1 at 2 months; DPT-2 at 4 months; DPT-3 at 6 months; OPV-1 at 2 months; OPV-2 at 4 months; OPV-3 at 6 months; measles at 9 months; BCG at birth and at 6 years or older.

BIBLIOGRAPHY

Adler MW, editor: Statistics from the World Health Organization and the Centers for Disease Control, *AIDS* 6(10):1229, 1992.

Holmes P: Diary from Honduras, *Nurs Times* 83(50):24, 1987.

Popkin BM et al: An evaluation of a national breast-feeding promotion programme in Honduras, *J Biosoc Sci* 23(1):5, 1991.

◆ HUNGARY

MAP PAGE (258)

Location: Hungary is a country of fertile rolling plains located in central Europe.

Major Languages	Ethnic Groups		Major Religions	
Hungarian	Magyar	97%	Catholic	68%
Other	German	2%	Calvinist	20%
	Gypsy and		Lutheran	5%
	Other	1%	Other	7%

Predominant Sick Care Practices: Biomedical.

Health Care Beliefs: Health promotion is important.

Ethnic/Race Specific or Endemic Diseases: RISK: Heart and lung diseases, such as cancer and tuberculosis.

Health Team Relationships: Nurses are subordinate to physicians.

Birth Rites: Hospital stay is 4 to 7 days; a health visitor is required to make a home visit within 24 hours after discharge.

Infant Feeding Practices: Breastfeeding is encouraged.

Child Rearing Practices: Children's health is monitored by health visitors until age 14.

National Childhood Immunizations: BCG between 3 and 42 days; DPT at 3 months, 4 months, 5 months, 36 months, and between 6 and 7 years; measles and rubella at 14 months; DT, measles, and rubella between 11 and 12 years.

BIBLIOGRAPHY

Arrindell WA et al: Cross-national generalizability of dimensions of perceived parental rearing practices: Hungary and the Netherlands: a correction and repetition with healthy adolescents, *Psychol Rep* 65(3 Part 2):1079, 1989.

Salvage J: Health in Hungary, *Senior Nurse* 5(1):27, 1986.

Solomon J: Critical care nursing, *Focus Crit Care* 13(3):10, 1986.

Trevelyan J: Taking the waters: natural thermal springs to treat a wide variety of ailments, *Nurs Times* 86(40):38, 1990.

◆ ICELAND

MAP PAGE (258)

Location: This north Atlantic island is Europe's most western point; it touches on the Arctic Circle. More than 13% is covered with snowfields and glaciers; it is one of the most volcanic regions in the world.

Major Language	Ethnic Groups		Major Religions	
Icelandic	Icelandish	99%	Lutheran	95%
	Other	1%	Other Christian	3%
			Unaffiliated and Other	2%

Ethnic/Race Specific or Endemic Diseases: Phenylketonuria.

Birth Rites: Almost all births occur in the hospital. Hospital stays range from 4 to 7 days. The semisitting position is common. The father and supportive individuals may be present. Normal deliveries are handled by midwives.

Infant Feeding Practices: Breastfeeding is common.

BIBLIOGRAPHY

Boyle JS, Andrews MM: *Transcultural concepts in nursing care,* Glenview, Ill, 1989, Scott, Foresman/Little, Brown College Division.

Einarsdottir ES: Midwifery education in Iceland, *J Nurse Midwifery* 28(6):31, 1983.

Paine LL, Palsdottir B: An American look at midwifery in Iceland, *J Nurse Midwifery* 32(5):319, 1987.

◆ INDIA

MAP PAGE (264)

Location: The world's most populous democracy extends from the Bay of Bengal on the east to the Arabian Sea on the west. India's three great river systems, the Ganges, Indus, and Brahmaputra, all have extensive deltas.

Major Languages	Ethnic Groups		Major Religions	
Hindi	Indo-Aryan	72%	Hindu	83%
English	Dravidian	25%	Muslim	11%
Other	Mongol		Christian	2%
	and Other	3%	Sikh	2%
			Buddhist	
			and Other	2%

Predominant Sick Care Practices: Biomedical; traditional. Spiritual values permeate most aspects of life and death. Allopathic medicine may be used in almost all rural communities. The poorer use more informal or traditional systems of medicine.

Health Care Beliefs: Acute sick care only. Diseases are believed to be caused by an upset in body balance.

Ethnic/Race Specific or Endemic Diseases: ACTIVE: Cholera. ENDEMIC: Chloroquine-resistant malaria. RISK: Japanese encephalitis; schistosomiasis.

Health Team Relationships: Some women object to being examined by a male physician. Terminal illness is not discussed with the patient by health care professionals; however, it may be discussed with the patient's relatives. Adults will not enter into the decision-making process if elderly parents are present. Nurses may not be able to influence health care decisions of patients and may work under medical or nontechnical personnel.

Dominance Patterns: Unquestioned obedience to elders is expected. A male child is especially desired. Women are dependent on men at every stage of life in traditional families; however, increased education and decision-making for some women are reported.

Touch Practices: Men may shake hands with other men but not with women. Instead, the man places his palms together and bows slightly. Bare upper arms or shoulders are considered indecent.

Time Perceptions: Minimal future time perspective is demonstrated. People are more oriented to the past. The concept of time is closely allied with an infinite universe of unending cycles that extend beyond birth, life, and death.

Pain Reactions: The patient has a quiet acceptance of pain and will accept some relief measures.

Birth Rites: Voluntary sterilization in males is encouraged, with monetary incentives and prizes. Amniocentesis may be used to determine the sex of the fetus, with possible abortion for a female. Cravings during pregnancy are satisfied because they are thought to be those of the fetus. Celebration of the birth of a son may include the beating of drums or blowing of conch shells. The midwife is paid a reward.

Death Rites: Hindu patients may make indirect references to their own deaths, often accepting God's will. The patient's desire to be clearheaded as death approaches must be assessed in planning medical treatment. Provision of time and place for prayer is essential for the family and patient; prayer helps deal with anxiety and conflict. The Hindu priest or anyone present may read from the Holy Sanskrit books. Some priests tie strings (signifying a blessing) around the neck or wrist and, after death, pour water into the mouth of the deceased. Families may prefer that non-Hindus not touch the body and may wash the body themselves. Blood transfusions, organ transplants, and autopsies are permitted. Cremation is preferred. Reincarnation is a Hindu belief.

Food Practices and Intolerances: Beef is not eaten.

Infant Feeding Practices: Breastfeeding on demand is the norm and is supplemented with other foods between 6 months and 1 year; however, breastfeeding may continue up to 3 years.

Child Rearing Practices: The predominant theme in child rearing is protective nurturing. The child is indulged, cuddled, and held and remains intimately and strongly attached to its mother until age 3 or 4. The toddler is not pushed into toilet training. The female's childhood is shorter because domestic responsibilities occur early. Discipline in late childhood includes scolding and light spanking. Children are rarely praised for doing what is expected of them; praise may bring on the evil eye.

National Childhood Immunizations: BCG at birth; DPT at 6 weeks, 10 weeks, and 14 weeks; booster at 16 months; DT booster at 5 years; TT booster at 10 and 16 years; measles at 9 months; OPV at 6 weeks, 10 weeks, and 14 weeks; OPV booster at 16 months.

Other Characteristics: Mortality statistics are higher for women than men, possibly because males receive preferential treatment. The Sikh religion forbids cutting or shaving any body hair. Older women enjoy a heightened social prestige. No expression for "thanks" exists; a social act is a fulfillment of an obligation or duty, requiring no verbal acknowledgment. The motions of the head for "yes" and "no" are opposite those in the United States.

BIBLIOGRAPHY

Ahmad WI: Patients' choice of general practitioner: intolerance of patients' fluency in English and the ethnicity and sex of the doctor, *J R Coll Gen Pract* 39(321):153, 1989.

Basu AM: Cultural influences on health care use: two regional groups in India, *Stud Fam Plann* 21(5):275, 1990.

Clark MJ: *Nursing in the community,* Norwalk, Conn, 1992, Appleton & Lange.

Condon JC, Yousef F: *An introduction to intercultural communication,* New York, 1975, Macmillan.

Davis CF: Culturally responsive nursing management in an international health care setting, *Nurs Admin Q* 16(2):36, 1992.

Dickson GL: The metalanguage of menopause research, *Image* 22(3):168, 1990.

Discovery Channel: A planet for the taking, March 15, 1989.

Fisher P: Chinese population crises. Unpublished paper, SOC 107W, University of Connecticut, 1989.

Francis MR: Concerns of terminally ill adult Hindu cancer patients, *Cancer Nurs* 9(4):164, 1986.

Galanti GA: *Caring for patients from different cultures,* Philadelphia, 1991, University of Pennsylvania Press.

Green J: Hinduism, *Nurs Times* 85(6):50, 1989.

Irujo S: *An introduction to intercultural differences and similarities in nonverbal communication.* In Wurzel JS, editor: *Toward multiculturalism,* Yarmouth, Me, 1988, Intercultural Press.

Izhar N: Patient origins and usage of a Unani clinic in Aligarh Town, India, *Soc Sci Med* 30(10):1139, 1990.

Kakar S: *The child in India.* In Wurzel JS, editor: *Toward multiculturalism,* Yarmouth, Me, 1988, Intercultural Press.

Lally MM: Last rites and funeral customs of minority groups, *Midwife Health Visit Comm Nurse* 14(7):224, 1978.

Marchione J, Stearns SJ: Ethnic power perspectives for nursing, *Nurs Health Care* 11(6):296, 1990.

Meade RD: Future time perspectives of Americans and subcultures in India, *J Cross-cult Psychol* 3(1):93, 1972.

Patel NR: Nursing in India, *Nurs Admin Q* 16(2):72, 1992.

Ramachandran H, Shastri GS: Movement for medical treatment: a study in contact patterns of a rural population, *Soc Sci Med* 17(3):177, 1983.

Samovar LA, Porter RE: *Intercultural communication: a reader,* Belmont, Calif, 1985, Wadsworth.

Sleed J: Manners abroad need study, Newhouse News Service.

Stewart EC, Bennett MJ: *American cultural patterns: a cross-cultural perspective,* rev ed, Yarmouth, Me, 1991, Intercultural Press.

Storti C: *The art of crossing cultures,* Yarmouth, Me, 1990, Intercultural Press.

Ullrich ME: A study of change and depression among Havik Brahmin women in a south Indian village, *Cult Med Psychiatry* 11(3):261, 1987.

Weisfeld GE: Sociobiological patterns of Arab culture, *Ethnol Sociobiol* 11:23, 1990.

◆ INDONESIA

MAP PAGE (265)

Location: Part of the Malay archipelago along the equator in Southeast Asia, Indonesia consists of 13,677 islands; approximately 6000 are inhabited. With mountains and plateaus the major islands have a cooler climate than the tropical lowlands.

Major Languages	Ethnic Groups		Major Religions	
Indonesian	Javanese	45%	Muslim	88%
English	Sundanese	14%	Protestant	6%
Dutch	Madurese	8%	Catholic	3%
Javanese	Coastal Malay	8%	Hindu	2%
	Other	25%	Other	1%

Predominant Sick Care Practices: Magico-religious. Belief in ancestor spirits, who are engaged in all aspects of life, is widespread. The *adat* (the way of the ancestors) governs rituals performed at births and funerals, as well as many other aspects of behavior.

Ethnic/Race Specific or Endemic Diseases: ACTIVE: Cholera. ENDEMIC: Chloroquine-resistant malaria, with no risk in major cities. RISK: Japanese encephalitis; schistosomiasis.

Health Team Relationships: Clients may consider titles more important than names.

Dominance Patterns: The roles of men and women are defined in the Koran, with women having limited possibilities.

Eye Contact Practices: Looking someone in the eye, especially for a woman, is improper and disrespectful.

Birth Rites: Having many children is valued. Children are the support of and a source of security for their parents in old age. Free birth control methods are available from the government and are distributed through health stations and in small shops.

Death Rites: Muslim belief forbids organ donation or transplants. Muslim physicians may recommend transfusions to save lives. Autopsy is uncommon because the deceased must be buried intact. Cremation is not permitted. For Muslim burial the body is wrapped in special pieces of cloth and buried without a coffin in the ground.

Food Practices and Intolerances: Pork, carrion, and blood are forbidden. During Ramadan, the Islamic month of fasting, breakfast has to be eaten before dawn, followed by a ritual washing to prepare for morning prayer, which must coincide with sunrise. During the day, eating or drinking is forbidden, with exceptions for children, the elderly, and the sick. At dusk, after the fourth ritual prayer of the day, the time for fasting is concluded.

National Childhood Immunizations: BCG at birth; three DPT at 4-week intervals between 2 months and 18 months; measles at 9 months; three OPV at 4-week intervals between 2 months and 18 months. World Health Organization universal immunization coverage standards are reported as achieved.

Other Characteristics: Men are allowed to have up to four wives at the same time. Carrying on a conversation with hands in the pockets is not received well; hands on the hips is perceived as defiance. The gesture of curling the index finger inward is used to call animals only.

BIBLIOGRAPHY

Hamke K, Kievelitz U: *Climbing the intercultural ladder: the gradual adaptation process to a village culture in Indonesia,* New York, 1986, AFS International/Intercultural Programs.

Paige RM: Formal education and psychosocial modernity in East Java, Indonesia, *Inter J Intercult Relations* 3:333, 1979.

Ross HM: Societal/cultural views regarding death and dying, *Top Clin Nurs* 1(1):1, 1981.

Samovar LA, Porter RE: *Intercultural communication: a reader,* Belmont, Calif, 1985, Wadsworth.

U.S. Agency for International Development: Indonesia lowers infant mortality, *Front Lines* 31(10):16, 1991.

Wikan U: Bereavement and loss in two Muslim communities: Egypt and Bali compared, *Soc Sci Med* 27(5):451, 1988.

◆ IRAN

MAP PAGE (262)

Location: This ancient land of Persia is an Islamic republic in the oil-rich Middle East. Although much is desert, there are oases, maritime lowlands along the Persian Gulf, and the Caspian Sea and mountains in the north. The populated areas are in the north and northwest. Iranians are stereotyped as Arabs; however, the Iranian language and culture are similar in some areas but different in others.

Major Languages	Ethnic Groups		Major Religions	
Farsi	Persian	63%	Shi'a Muslim	93%
Turkish	Turkish	18%	Sunni Muslim	5%
Kurdish	Kurdish	3%	Bahai and	
Arabic	Arab and		Other	2%
English	Other	16%		

Predominant Sick Care Practices: Biomedical; magico-religious. Various beliefs in the causes of disease coexist, such as the hot/cold humoral theory and the evil eye. A physically robust person is considered healthier. Emotional distress, especially fear, anger and grief, may be expressed as "heart distress" with irregular cardiac rate.

Health Care Beliefs: Acute sick care only. Medications by injection may be preferred. Patients who do not receive a written prescription may believe that the physician did not properly treat them.

Ethnic/Race Specific or Endemic Diseases: ENDEMIC: Chloroquine-resistant malaria, with no risk in urban areas. RISK: Schistosomiasis.

Health Team Relationships: The physician's authority is not questioned; the patient and family may not ask questions or give any information that might be construed as disrespectful. The reason for personal questions during assessment needs to be made clear to the patient. Males may refuse care by female physicians and nurses. Aggressiveness, toughness, and even pushiness are acceptable behaviors for ensuring good care.

Families' Role in Hospital Care: A patient may be accompanied by one or more persons who wish to be present during examination, answering questions for the patient. The eldest person present must be included in the discussion. The family role is fulfilled by demanding behavior and extreme concern and attention. Repetition in communication is commonly used for emphasis and to indicate the importance of the matter.

Dominance Patterns: It is a patriarchal society. Children are expected to submit to the authority of the father. The family and their position in society predominate, rather than the individual.

Eye Contact Practices: A woman making direct eye contact with a man implies promiscuity and an interest in dating.

Touch Practices: Touch is frequent, as are closeness and embracing on arrival and departure.

Time Perceptions: Punctuality is not important; establishing a relationship before talking business is more important.

Pain Reactions: The Iranian woman may yell throughout labor. The custom is to compensate a woman for her suffering during childbirth by giving her gifts.

Birth Rites: Restrictions do not exist during pregnancy. A suspected pregnancy may not be announced, even to the father. Women may shave their bodies in preparation for childbirth. Birth occurs at home, especially in rural villages. The husband is not present but may be nearby. Males are circumcised anytime after birth until age 5. Dietary restrictions may be in effect for 40 days after the birth.

Death Rites: Impending death is concealed from the patient by any means possible. Muslim belief forbids organ donations or transplants. Muslim physicians may recommend transfusions to save lives. A Holy Iman does not have to be present at death. A Muslim should help the patient or recite the Declaration of the Faith: "There is no God but God, and Muhammed is his Messenger." Grief is not permitted in the dying person's presence. After death, family members wash the body, according to Islamic tradition, before the funeral. Once death has occurred, mourning is loud, obvious, and expressive. Autopsy is uncommon because the deceased must be buried intact, without embalming or a casket. Cremation is not permitted.

Food Practices and Intolerances: The main meal is at midday. Islamic law does not permit the consumption of pork, alcohol, or meat that has not been slaughtered according to the Islamic code. In poorer families the male may receive the most nutritious food. Ramadan fasting is observed between sunrise and sunset, with exemptions for children and the sick.

Infant Feeding Practices: Pacifiers are acceptable. Weaning may be abrupt at age 2 years. Supplementary foods are given beginning at 4 to 5 months.

Child Rearing Practices: Fathers have greater control of resources and have the authoritarian power, while mothers exert greater control in child nurturing and value transmission. Belief dictates that excessive praise of a child may cast the evil eye. Toilet training may begin as early as 3 months. Traditional girls wear the veil at age 7 or earlier. Girls are taught to look straight ahead and never to look at men when they are outside. Boys and girls no longer play together after age 5. Discipline of male children is limited.

National Childhood Immunizations: OPV at birth; OPV-1 at 2 months; OPV-2 at 4 months; OPV-3 at 6 months.

Other Characteristics: The U.S. finger gestures for thumbs up and the V are insulting. Distance kept during conversation is close.

BIBLIOGRAPHY

Boyle JS, Andrews MM: *Transcultural concepts in nursing care,* Glenview, Ill, 1989, Scott, Foresman/Little, Brown College Division.

Galanti GA: *Caring for patients from different cultures,* Philadelphia, 1991, University of Pennsylvania Press.

Green J: Death with dignity: Islam, *Nurs Times* 85(5):56, 1989.

Kendall K: Maternal and child care in an Iranian village, *J Transcult Nurs* 3(1):29, 1992.

Lally MM: Last rites and funeral customs of minority groups, *Midwife Health Visit Comm Nurse* 14(7):224, 1978.

Lipson JG, Meleis AI: Issues in health care of Middle Eastern patients, *West Med J* 139(6):854, 1983.

Luna LJ: Transcultural nursing: care of Arab Muslims, *J Transcult Nurs* 1(1):22, 1989.

Meleis AI, LaFever CW: The Arab American psychiatric care, *Perspect Psychiatr Care* 22(2):72, 1984.

Ross HM: Societal/cultural views regarding death and dying, *Top Clin Nurs* 1(1):1, 1981.

Spector RE: *Cultural diversity in health and illness,* ed 3, Norwalk, Conn, 1991, Appleton & Lange.

Stewart EC, Bennett MJ: *American cultural patterns: a cross-cultural perspective,* rev ed, Yarmouth, Me, 1991, Intercultural Press.

Tashakkori A, Thompson VD: Effects of family configuration variables on reported indices of parental power among Iranian adolescents, *Soc Biol* 35(1-2):82, 1988.

◆ IRAQ

MAP PAGE (262)

Location: Iraq occupies the valley between the Tigris and Euphrates rivers. Mountains are set in the north and desert in the southwest, with marshland along the Persian Gulf.

Major Languages	Ethnic Groups		Major Religions	
Arabic	Arab	75%	Shi'a Muslim	62%
Kurdish	Kurdish	17%	Sunni Muslim	35%
Assyrian	Other	8%	Christian and	
Armenian			Other	3%

Ethnic/Race Specific or Endemic Diseases: ENDEMIC: Chloroquine-sensitive malaria. RISK: Schistosomiasis.

Health Team Relationships: The reason for asking the patient personal questions during assessment needs to be made clear. Males may refuse care by female physicians and nurse practitioners. Nursing is a female profession with low status and with a negative image.

Families' Role in Hospital Care: A patient may be accompanied by one or more persons who wish to be present during examination and answer questions for the patient. The eldest person present expects to be included in the discussion. The family role is fulfilled through demanding behavior and extreme concern and attention.

Dominance Patterns: It is a patriarchal society. Sexual inequities are part of the legal system that relegates women to an inferior status. However, women exercise power in the domestic arena.

Touch Practices: Touch, closeness, and embracing on arrival and departure, are common.

Time Perceptions: The society is oriented to the present because planning ahead may defy God's will. Punctuality is not important; establishing a relationship before talking business is more important.

Pain Reactions: Pain relief is expected to be immediate and may be requested persistently. Therapies requiring exertion contraindicate the people's belief in energy conservation for recovery. Pain is expressed privately or only with close relatives and friends. However, during labor and delivery, pain may be expressed vehemently.

Death Rites: Muslim belief forbids organ donations or transplants. Muslim physicians may recommend transfusions to save lives. Autopsy is uncommon because the deceased must be buried intact. Cremation is not permitted. For Muslim burial the body is wrapped in special pieces of cloth and buried without a coffin in the ground.

Food Practices and Intolerances: Pork, carrion, and blood are forbidden. Food tends to be spicy. Ramadan fasting is practiced between sunrise and sunset, with exemptions for children and the sick.

Child Rearing Practices: A government-sponsored fertility campaign encourages families to have at least five children.

National Childhood Immunizations: OPV-1 at 2 months; OPV-2 at 4 months; OPV-3 at 6 months.

Other Characteristics: Hope, optimism, and the positive advantages of treatment need to be stressed. Negative effects and outcomes should be minimized.

BIBLIOGRAPHY

Boyle JS: Professional nursing in Iraq, *Image* 21(3):168, 1989.

Green J: Death with dignity: Islam, *Nurs Times* 85(5):56, 1989.

Meleis AI, LaFever CW: The Arab American and psychiatric care, *Perspect Psychiatr Care* 22(2):72, 1984.

Meleis AI, Sorrell L: Arab American women and their birth experiences, *MCN* 6:171, 1981.

Reizian A, Meleis AI: Arab-Americans' perceptions of and responses to pain, *Crit Care Nurse* 6(6):30, 1986.

Ross HM: Societal/cultural views regarding death and dying, *Top Clin Nurs* 1(1):1, 1981.

◆ IRELAND

MAP PAGE (258)

Location: Ireland, an island country in the Atlantic Ocean, is separated from Britain by the Irish Sea. It is generally bowl shaped, with a central plain surrounded by low mountains; the highest peak is 3415 feet (1041 m).

Major Languages	Ethnic Groups		Major Religions	
Irish (Gaelic)	Irish	99%	Catholic	94%
English	Other	1%	Anglican	4%
			Other	2%

Ethnic/Race Specific or Endemic Diseases: **RISK:** Phenylketonuria; neural tube defects; high mortality from coronary heart disease.

Pain Reactions: The Irish are typically inexpressive and stoic; they do not vocalize pain and are less apt to describe pain as extremely intense. They prefer company but will try to hide pain from family and friends. The desire to be alone after freely admitting pain is also possible.

Death Rites: The practice of watching or "waking" the dead originates from keeping vigil to keep evil spirits away from the deceased; it has become a religious ritual.

National Childhood Immunizations: BCG at birth and at 12 to 14 years for nonreactors; DPT at 3 months, 4½ months and 8½ months; DT at 5 years; TOPV at 3 months, 4½ months, 8½ months, and 5 years; MMR at 15 months; rubella between 10 and 14 years.

BIBLIOGRAPHY

Boyle JS, Andrews MM: *Transcultural concepts in nursing care,* Glenview, Ill, 1989, Scott, Foresman/Little, Brown College Division.

Broach J, Newton N: Food and beverages in labor, Part 1, cross-cultural and historical practices, *Birth* 15(2):81, 1988.

Galanti GA: *Caring for patients from different cultures,* Philadelphia, 1991, University of Pennsylvania Press.

Lipton JA, Marbach JJ: Ethnicity and the pain experience, *Soc Sci Med* 19(12):1279, 1984.

Martinelli AM: Pain and ethnicity: how people of different cultures experience pain, *AORN J* 46(2):273, 1987.

Shelley E et al: The Kilkenny Health Project: a community research and demonstration cardiovascular health programme, *Ir J Med Sci Suppl* 160(9):10, 1991.

Spector RE: *Cultural diversity in health and illness,* ed 3, Norwalk, Conn, 1991, Appleton & Lange.

Stone FA: *The Irish in their homeland, in America, in Connecticut,* Storrs, 1975, World Education Project, School of Education, University of Connecticut.

◆ ISRAEL

MAP PAGE (262)

Location: Formerly Palestine, Israel is located at the eastern end of the Mediterranean Sea. The coastal plain is fertile, and the southern region is primarily desert.

Major Languages	Ethnic Groups		Major Religions	
Hebrew	Jewish	83%	Jewish	83%
Arabic	Arab and		Muslim	13%
English	Other	17%	Christian	2%
French			Druze	2%

Health Care Beliefs: Passive role. A tendency toward passivity exists, and health self-care is not prevalent. Religion is part of daily life. Orthodox Jews may prefer not to travel, write, or turn on electrical appliances on the Sabbath.

Ethnic/Race Specific or Endemic Diseases: RISK: Infantile Tay-Sachs disease; infantile Niemann-Pick disease; adult Gaucher disease; Mediterranean fever.

Health Team Relationships: Assertiveness and toughness are acceptable behaviors.

Touch Practices: Touching is demonstrative.

Time Perceptions: Orientation toward the present is continuous, while future orientation decreases and past orientation increases with age.

Pain Reactions: Expressive, loud reactions may serve to communicate distress or call for reassurance, especially with chronic pain. People are more likely to blame themselves for pain. They hide pain from family and friends and are not inclined to describe the details of pain.

Death Rites: Before death a fatal prognosis is usually not discussed between the patient and family members. Chrysanthemums are used for funerals. Survivors' grief can be eased if the health care professional provides a biomedical explanation for the cause of death and reiterates the inevitability of death.

National Childhood Immunizations: DT/DPT at 3 months and 4 to 6 months; DPT between 5 and 7 months; DT between 11 and 13 months and 5 and 7 years; OPV or IPV at 3 months, between 4 and 6 months, 5 and 7 months, and 11 and 13 months, and at 3 years. Hepatitis B at 3 months and between 4 and 6 months and 11 and 13 months from positive mothers; measles between 11 and 13 months; rubella for girls and mumps for boys between 9 and 12 years.

Other Characteristics: The gesture for "no" is palm up, with the fingers curling inwards and moving back and forth.

BIBLIOGRAPHY

Boyle JS, Andrews MM: *Transcultural concepts in nursing care,* Glenview, Ill, 1989, Scott, Foresman/Little, Brown College Division.

Eisenbruch M: Cross-cultural aspects of bereavement. II. Ethnic and cultural variations in the development of bereavement practices, *Cult Med Psychiatry* 8(4):315, 1984.

Galanti GA: *Caring for patients from different cultures,* Philadelphia, 1991, University of Pennsylvania Press.

Giger JN, Davidhizar RE: *Transcultural nursing,* St Louis, 1991, Mosby.

Lipton JA, Marbach JJ: Ethnicity and the pain experience, *Soc Sci Med* 19(12):1279, 1984.

Martinelli AM: Pain and ethnicity: how people of different cultures experience pain, *AORN J* 46(2):273, 1987.

Migliore S: Punctuality, pain and time-orientation among Sicilian-Canadians, *Soc Sci Med* 28(8):851, 1989.

Ragucci AT: *Italian Americans.* In Harwood A, editor: *Ethnicity and medical care,* Cambridge, Mass, 1981, Harvard University Press.

Ross HM: Societal/cultural views regarding death and dying, *Top Clin Nurs* 1(1):1, 1981.

Spector RE: *Cultural diversity in health and illness,* ed 3, Norwalk, Conn, 1991, Appleton & Lange.

Stewart EC, Bennett MJ: *American cultural patterns: a cross-cultural perspective,* rev ed, Yarmouth, Me, 1991, Intercultural Press.

◆ IVORY COAST (CÔTE D'IVOIRE)

MAP PAGE (260)

Location: The Ivory Coast is located on the western African coast along the Gulf of Guinea. Rainfall is heavy along the coastline; dense forests are prevalent in the interior and savannas in the north. The Ivory Coast is one of the most stable and prosperous countries in tropical Africa.

Major Languages	Ethnic Groups		Major Religions	
French	Baoule	23%	Indigenous	
Diola	Bete	18%	Beliefs	63%
Other	Senoufou	15%	Muslim	25%
	Malinke	11%	Christian	12%
	Other	33%		

Predominant Sick Care Practices: Magico-religious; traditional. Basic concepts of Western medicine may not be known.

Health Care Beliefs: Acute sick care.

Ethnic/Race Specific or Endemic Diseases: ACTIVE: Cholera. ENDEMIC: Yellow fever; chloroquine-resistant malaria. RISK: Schistosomiasis. AIDS case rate is 26.6/ 100,000 people.

Infant Feeding Practices: Breastfed infants are weaned at 10 months. Breastfeeding is done openly.

Child Rearing Practices: Herbal enemas are given to neonates.

National Childhood Immunizations: BCG at birth; DPT-1 at 2 months; DPT-2 at 3 months; DPT-3 at 4 months; DPT booster at 17 to 18 months; DT at 6 to 7 years; measles at 9 months; OPV-1 at 2 months; OPV-2 at 3 months; OPV-3 at 4 months; OPV booster at 17 to 18 months.

BIBLIOGRAPHY

Abdel-Al H: Upper Volta and Ivory Coast: responding to nurses' needs, *Int Nurs Rev* 30(3):87, 1983.

Adler MW, editor: Statistics from the World Health Organization and the Centers for Disease Control, *AIDS* 6(10):1229, 1992.

Lobb M: An American nurse visits a M & CW clinic in West Africa, *Int Nurs Rev* 30(6):175, 1983.

♦ JAMAICA

MAP PAGE (257)

Location: This island nation is located 90 miles (145 km) south of Cuba in the West Indies of the Caribbean.

Major Languages	Ethnic Groups		Major Religions	
English	African	76%	Protestant	55%
Creole	Afro-		Catholic	20%
	European	15%	Spiritualist	20%
	Afro-Asian	4%	Other	5%
	White	3%		
	Other	2%		

Many Jamaicans are born of English-African sexual unions.

Predominant Sick Care Practices: Biomedical; magico-religious. Traditional healers coexist in conjunction with modern medicine.

Health Care Beliefs: Health promotion is important.

Dominance Patterns: The trend is matrifocal: women having independence. Having a lifetime partner is not important; therefore several different fathers may visit with their children in one household.

Time Perceptions: Rewards for current activity are preferred over delayed gratification.

Birth Rites: Traditional practices may include smelling the perspiration on the father's shirt to speed labor.

Infant Feeding Practices: Even though the rate of infant mortality caused by malnutrition is high, breastfeeding is declining, especially after age 3 months. Carbohydrate gruels, porridge, fruit juices, and herbal teas are bottle fed at an early age. Mothers from urban middle income groups terminate breastfeeding earlier than lower income mothers.

Child Rearing Practices: Mothers often live in an extended family or live alone with their children. Infants are often carried and can suckle on demand. Control over aggressive behavior is encouraged.

National Childhood Immunizations: No data located.

Other Characteristics: Diarrhea is called "runny belly," and vitamins are referred to as "tonic." A love of music and dance are deep cultural values and may be used as vehicles for conveying health concepts.

BIBLIOGRAPHIES

Bailey KM: Cross cultural experience in Jamaica, *Maine Nurse* 75(20):6, 1989.

Bates B, Turner AN: Imagery and symbolism in the birth practices of traditional cultures, *Birth* 12(1):29, 1985.

Cunningham WC, Segree W: Breast feeding promotion in an urban and a rural Jamaican hospital, *Soc Sci Med* 30(3):341, 1990.

Dechesnay M: Jamaican family structure: the paradox of normalcy, *Fam Proc* 25:293, 1986.

Giugliani ERJ, Lovel H, Ebrahim GJ: Attitudes, practices and knowledge of health professionals on breast feeding in Kingston, Jamaica, *J Trop Pediatr* 34(4):169, 1988.

Green HB: Temporal attitudes in four Negro subcultures, *Studium Generale* 23(6):571, 1970.

Lambert MC, Weisz JR, Knight F: Over- and undercontrolled clinic referral problems of Jamaican and American children and adolescents: the culture general and the culture specific, *J Consult Clin Psychol* 57(4):467, 1989.

Mason C: Women as mothers in Northern Ireland and Jamaica: a critique of the transcultural nursing movement, *Int J Nurs Stud* 27(4):367, 1990.

Standard KL, Minott OD: A song and a dance, *World Health* Apr-May:5, 1983.

Stewart EC, Bennett MJ: *American cultural patterns: a cross-cultural perspective,* rev ed, Yarmouth, Me, 1991, Intercultural Press.

◆ **JAPAN**

MAP PAGE (263)

Location: A Pacific Ocean archipelago, Japan extends 1744 miles (2790 km) and is separated from the east coast of Asia by the Sea of Japan. The main islands have mountains separated by narrow fissures and valleys.

Major Language	Ethnic Groups		Major Religions	
Japanese	Japanese	99%	Shinto Buddhist	84%
	Korean	1%	Other	16%

Predominant Sick Care Practices: Magico-religious. Consultation with priests to seek luck and avoid evil may precede important activities or decisions.

Health Care Beliefs: Physical diseases are placed in the context of the patient's social relations.

Ethnic/Race Specific or Endemic Diseases: RISK: Japanese encephalitis; schistosomiasis; acatalasemia; cleft lip or palate; Oguchi disease.

Health Team Relationships: Respect for social rank is pervasive. The physician is expected to know best and use good judgment; consent forms are not generally used. Deference to caregivers' authority results in few questions being asked. Questions involving a "no" answer often fail to get an accurate answer or needed information. "I'll do my best" is a polite way of declining. Titles are important; they may be used rather than the names of caregivers. Patterns of thought are expressed indirectly with the listener expected to get the point without being explicitly told. Asking the question "What" is preferred. Increasingly refined details will be uncovered with each question. The patient may divert the subject away from an embarrassing topic or avoid direct confrontation. Patient complaints may be made by a third-party mediator or may be indirectly indicated by the patient. Individual verbal agreement does not mean compliance. When medical decisions are made, the family is consulted first.

Families' Role in Hospital Care: Family interdependence takes precedence over independence; therefore self-care is not an important concept. Family participation in care is expected. The patient's mother or someone else gives personal care 24 hours a day.

Dominance Patterns: Women are traditionally passive and domesticated. The woman has power in rearing children, in family budgeting, and in achieving success in school. Parents expect to be cared for in their old age. Many of these traditional patterns are changing in today's Japan.

Eye Contact Practices: Direct eye contact is considered a lack of respect and a personal affront. Preference is for the "lighthouse" sweep, shifting, or downcast eyes.

Touch Practices: Handshakes are acceptable; however, a pat on the back is not. A kiss may show deference to superiors.

Time Perceptions: Promptness is valued.

Pain Reactions: Patients stoically withstand discomfort.

Birth Rites: Japan has one of the lowest infant mortality rates in the industrialized world. Premature birth weight is suggested at 2300 g. The people comply with prenatal care and health promotion readily. Women labor in silence and eat more food during labor. After delivery, long periods of rest and recuperation are practiced. The mother may remain indoors for as long as 100 days; she may not wish to bathe or wash her hair for a week.

Death Rites: A smile that expresses the desire not to have others worry about a personal bereavement may accompany the announcement or discussion of the death of a family member. The Japanese tend to control public expression of grief.

Food Practices and Intolerances: Raw fish is eaten.

Infant Feeding Practices: Although early breastfeeding is almost universal, only half of babies are breastfed after 1 month. Colostrum is not fed to the newborn.

Child Rearing Practices: The mother/child relationship is strong. The mother may sleep with her child or watch vigilantly while the child sleeps. Respect for authority figures and collaborative decision making are taught. Boys may be socialized to be assertive and successful in their achievements. Girls are taught to enjoy life and suppress ideas. Students spend long hours preparing for university entrance examinations. This period is highly stressful in the child's life.

National Childhood Immunizations: DPT at 3 months; 3¾ months, and 4½ months; DPT booster at 1½ years; DT at 11 years; polio at 3 months and 4½ months; BCG at 3 months, 6 years, and 13 years; measles at 1 year; rubella for girls at junior high school age.

Other Characteristics: Fever is treated by sweating it out, using warm blankets, and drinking hot drinks. As a sign of social politeness, the Japanese hiss, a sudden breathing inward. Laughter is a common sign of embarrassment, masks bereavement, and conceals rage; happiness is masked with a straight face. The Japanese do not rinse themselves in the same water in which they have bathed. Bathing usually occurs just before bedtime; however, it is suspended during times of illness. The lower and longer the greeting bow, with the head and eyes lowered, the more respect shown.

BIBLIOGRAPHIES

Bennett MJ: *Towards ethnorelativism: a developmental model of intercultural sensitivity.* In Paige RM: *Cross-cultural orientation: new conceptualizations and applications,* Lanham, Md, 1986, University Press of America.

Boyle JS, Andrews MM: *Transcultural concepts in nursing care,* Glenview, Ill, 1989, Scott, Foresman/Little, Brown College Division.

Condon JC, Yousef F: *An introduction to intercultural communication,* New York, 1975, Macmillan.

Connor JW: Kankei J: A key concept for an understanding of Japanese-American achievement, *Psychiatry* 39(3):266, 1976.

Eisenbruch M: Cross-cultural aspects of bereavement, II, ethnic and cultural variations in the development of bereavement practices, *Culture Med Psychiatry* 8(4):315, 1984.

Engel NS: An American experience of pregnancy and childbirth in Japan, *Birth* 16(2):81, 1989.

Galanti GA: *Caring for patients from different cultures,* Philadelphia, 1991, University of Pennsylvania Press.

Grove CL: *Communications across cultures,* Washington, DC, 1976, National Education Association.

Kagawa-Singer M: Ethnic perspectives of cancer nursing: Hispanics and Japanese-Americans, *Cancer Nurs Perspect* 14(3):59, 1987.

Kobayashi M: Promoting breast-feeding: a successful regional project in Japan, *Acta Paediatr Jpn* 31(4):404, 1989.

Lally MM: Last rites and funeral customs of minority groups, *Midwife Health Visit Comm Nurse* 14(7):224, 1978.

Lock MM: Scars of experience: the art of moxibustion in Japanese medicine and society, *Cult Med Psychiatry* 2(2):151, 1978.

Myano Y: Personal communication, July 25, 1991.

Overfield T: *Biologic variation in health and illness,* Menlo Park, Calif, 1985, Addison-Wesley.

Prosser MH: *The cultural dialogue,* Washington, DC, 1985, SIETAR.

Pusch MD, editor: *Multicultural education,* Yarmouth, Me, 1981, Intercultural Press.

Shand N: Culture's influence in Japanese and American maternal role perception and confidence, *Psychiatry* 48(1):52, 1985.

Sikkema M, Niyekawa A: *Design for cross-cultural learning,* Yarmouth, Me, 1987, Intercultural Press.

Sleed J: Manners abroad need study, Newhouse News Service, n.d.

Stewart EC, Danielian J, Foster RJ: *Stimulating intercultural communication through role-playing,* Portland, Ore, 1991 seminar handout, SIIC.

Stewart EC, Bennett MJ: *American cultural patterns: a cross-cultural perspective,* rev ed, Yarmouth, Me, 1991, Intercultural Press.

Storti C: *The art of crossing cultures,* Yarmouth, Me, 1990, Intercultural Press.

Trommsdorff G: Value change in Japan, *Int J Intercult Relations* 7:337, 1983.

Yamamoto J et al: Mourning in Japan, *Am J Psychiatry* 125(12):1660, 1969.

Yoshikawa M: *Some Japanese and American cultural characteristics.* In Prosser MH: *The cultural dialogue,* Washington, DC, 1985, SIETAR.

◆ JORDAN

MAP PAGE (262)

Location: Formerly Transjordan, Jordan is located in the Middle East. It is an arid country, with fertile areas only in the west.

Major Languages	Ethnic Groups		Major Religions	
Arabic	Arab	98%	Sunni Muslim	95%
English	Circassian	1%	Christian	5%
	Armenian	1%		

Predominant Sick Care Practices: Biomedical; magico-religious.

Health Care Beliefs: Acute sick care only. Health means the ability to function.

Health Team Relationships: The patient needs to know the reason for personal questions during assessment. Males may refuse care by female physicians or nurse practitioners. Approximately half the country's nurses are male.

Families' Role in Hospital Care: A patient may be accompanied by one or many family members, who wish to be present during examination and who may answer questions for the patient. Families may sleep and cook in the patient's room. The health care professional should include the eldest person present in discussions with the patient. The family may exhibit demanding behavior and show extreme concern toward and attention to the patient.

Dominance Patterns: It is a patriarchal society.

Eye Contact Practices: Direct eye contact is practiced in conversation; the listener frequently looks to the side.

Touch Practices: Handshaking is common; however, a traditionally dressed female may not shake hands with or touch a male. Handholding is practiced among the same sex.

Time Perceptions: Generally, this society is oriented in the present because planning ahead implies defying God's will. Punctuality is not as important as taking time to establish a relationship before talking business.

Pain Reactions: Pain relief is expected immediately and may be requested persistently. Therapies requiring exertion contraindicate the belief in energy conservation for recovery. Pain is expressed privately or in the company of close relatives or friends. During labor and delivery pain is expressed loudly.

Birth Rites: The mother may have a 40-day lying-in period after birth. Her mother or sisters care for the infant. Males are circumcised. Male infants are more valued than females. Traditionally, infants are rubbed with salt and oil and are swaddled immediately after delivery.

Death Rites: Muslim belief forbids organ donations or transplants. Muslim physicians may recommend transfusions to save lives. Autopsy is uncommon because the deceased must be buried intact. For Muslim burial the body is wrapped in special pieces of cloth and buried without a coffin in the ground. Cremation is not permitted.

Food Practices and Intolerances: Chicken and lamb are widely consumed. Pork, carrion, and blood are forbidden. Food tends to be spicy. Ramadan fasting is practiced between sunrise and sunset, with exemptions for the sick and for children.

National Childhood Immunizations: OPV-1 at 2 months; OPV-2 between 3 and 4 months; OPV-3 between 5 and 6 months; OPV boosters between 15 and 24 months and 6 and 8 years. Immunizations are believed to be curative, with limited understanding of their preventive purpose.

Other Characteristics: Some very traditional women wear veils, while others cover only their hair and still others wear casual Western dress. A close conversational distance (about 18 inches to 2 feet) is practiced. Hope, optimism, and the positive advantages of treatment should be stressed when discussing outcomes.

BIBLIOGRAPHY

Ahmad SW: Personal perceptions of health: a transcultural study of Jordanian and south western U.S. senior nursing students, A paper presented at the Second Annual Middle East Nursing Conference, Irbid, Jordan, Apr 1992.

Beardslee C et al: Nursing care of children in developing countries: issues in Thailand, Botswana and Jordan, *Rec Adv Nurs* 16:31, 1987.

Geissler EM: Personal observations, April 23–May 4, 1992.

Green J: Death with dignity: Islam, *Nurs Times* 85(5):56, 1989.

Jafar E: Personal communication, Apr 28, 1992, Irbid, Jordan.

Khalaf IA: The relationship between the type of the child's death whether anticipated or unexpected and the Jordanian mother's grief responses. Doctoral dissertation, New York, 1989, New York University.

Lawson ED, Smadi OM, Tel SA: Values in Jordanian university students: a test of Osgood's cultural universals, *Int J Intercult Rel* 10:35, 1986.

Meleis AI, LaFever CW: The Arab American psychiatric care, *Perspect Psychiatr Care* 22(2):72, 1984.

Meleis AI, Sorrell L: Arab American women and their birth experiences, *MCN* 6:171, 1981.

Reizian A, Meleis AI: Arab-Americans' perceptions of and responses to pain, *Crit Care Nurse* 6(6):30, 1986.

Ross HM: Societal/cultural views regarding death and dying, *Top Clin Nurs* 1(1):1, 1981.

Sandford V: Nursing in the Middle East: a Jordan experience, *NZ Nurs J* 78(3):8, 1985.

◆ KENYA

MAP PAGE (261)

Location: Kenya is located on the equator on the east coast of Africa. Part of its border is on the Indian Ocean. Kenya is arid in the north. In the southwest corner lies the fertile Lake Victoria Basin. The Great Rift Valley, flanked by high mountains, extends north to south.

Major Languages	Ethnic Groups		Major Religions	
English	Kikuyu	21%	Protestant	38%
Swahili	Luhya	14%	Catholic	28%
Other	Luo	13%	Indigenous	
	Kalenjin	11%	Beliefs	26%
	Kamba		Muslim	8%
	and Other	41%		

Predominant Sick Care Practices: Biomedical; traditional. Herbalists often boil ingredients into tea.

Ethnic/Race Specific or Endemic Diseases: ENDEMIC: Yellow fever; chloroquine-resistant malaria. ACTIVE: Cholera. RISK: Schistosomiasis.

Pain Reactions: Pain relief measures are not common. Some believe that pain is necessary to become well again.

National Childhood Immunizations: BCG at birth; DPT-1 at 6 weeks; DPT-2 at 10 weeks; DPT-3 at 14 weeks; measles at 9 months; OPV at birth; OPV-1 at 6 weeks; OPV-2 at 10 weeks; OPV-3 at 14 weeks. Some do not understand the preventive nature of immunizations.

Other Characteristics: Nairobi women hold positions in business and, although not at high levels, in government offices. Birth control is strongly encouraged. Urban women place high value on maintaining a small family unit. Injections are preferred over tablets, and rectal medications may not be tolerated because the rectum is a taboo area of the body.

BIBLIOGRAPHY

Blair J: Health teaching in the context of culture: nursing in East Africa, *Kans Nurse* 66(4):4, 1991.

deVries MW, deVries MR: Cultural relativity of toilet training readiness: a perspective from East Africa, *Pediatrics* 60(2):170, 1977.

Jackson M, Morris S: An African adventure, *Nurs J Clin Pract Educ Manage* 4(21):28, 1990.

McInerney TG: Cross-cultural nursing: a perioperative experience in Kenya, *AORN J* 45(4):1000, 1987.

◆ KIRIBATI

MAP PAGE (255)

Location: Formerly the Gilbert Islands, Kiribati now includes 16 Gilbert Islands, eight Phoenix Islands, eight Line Islands, and Banaba. Located in the mid-Pacific, it is the largest atoll state in the world. Most islands are low lying with erratic rainfall.

Major Languages	Ethnic Groups		Major Religions	
English	Micronesian	99%	Catholic	48%
Gilbertese	Other	1%	Protestant	45%
			Other	7%

Ethnic/Race Specific or Endemic Diseases: RISK: Dengue fever; cholera.

Dominance Patterns: In this egalitarian society, boasting or elevating oneself above another is not acceptable.

Time Perceptions: Life moves at a slow and deliberate pace.

Food Practices and Intolerances: Breadfruit boiled or fried in butter is a staple. A great variety of fish is eaten.

National Childhood Immunizations: BCG at birth and at school entry; DPT at 3 months, 4 months, and 5 months; DPT booster at school entry; polio at 8 weeks, 10 weeks, and 14 weeks; measles at 9 months.

Other Characteristics: People are friendly, may appear embarrassingly bold, and are inquisitive about others. People squat to defecate; indoor toilet facilities are not readily available.

BIBLIOGRAPHY

Stanley D: *Micronesia handbook: guide to an American lake,* Chico, Calif, 1985, Moon.

◆ KOREA (NORTH)

MAP PAGE (263)

Location: The Democratic People's Republic of Korea occupies the northern part of the 600-mile (966 km) Korean peninsula off eastern Asia. Most of the country is covered with hills and north-to-south mountains; narrow valleys and small plains lie in between the mountains.

Major Language	Ethnic Groups		Major Religions	
Korean	Korean	99%	Atheist and	
	Other	1%	Unaffiliated	95%
			Buddhist and	
			Confucianism	5%

Health Team Relationships: A person's status and position are respected.

Families' Role in Hospital Care: Family interdependence takes precedence over independence, so self-care is not an important concept.

Touch Practices: Hand-holding and touching between friends of the same sex is accepted.

Time Perceptions: Continuing a social interaction is more important than being on time for another engagement.

Death Rites: Confucian funerals are elaborate rituals. After death and before burial, breakfast and supper are ceremoniously served to the deceased. A chief mourner and the relatives present weep.

Food Practices and Intolerances: In traditional families the father may dine alone using chopsticks or a spoon. After meals, which usually consist of rice, fish, soup, and vegetables, conversation ensues.

National Childhood Immunizations: BCG at 1 week and at 2, 5, 8, 12, 16, and 20 years; DPT at 3 months, 5 months, and 7 months; tetanus at 3 years and then at every 5 years; measles at 12 months and between 6 and 7 years and 16 and 17 years; OPV-1, 2, and 3 at 2- to 4-month intervals (starting age not stated); OPV boosters at 2, 3, 4, 5, 6, 8, and 10 years.

Other Characteristics: Both hands are used to transfer something to another person. The legs are not crossed during prayer and song at religious ceremonies. Sunglasses are removed when speaking with others. Males who urinate at the side of the road and children who run around without clothes are displaying acceptable behaviors. Names are placed in the following order: the family name first, generation name second, and personal or first name last. A woman does not change her name when she marries.

BIBLIOGRAPHY

Refer also to South Korea.
Galanti GA: *Caring for patients from different cultures,* Philadelphia, 1991, University of Pennsylvania Press.

◆ KOREA (SOUTH)

MAP PAGE (263)

Location: The Republic of Korea (South Korea) is located on a peninsula jutting from Manchuria and China off eastern Asia and below the 38th parallel. Eastern Korea is mountainous. The west and south have many mainland harbors and offshore islands.

Major Languages	Ethnic Groups		Major Religions	
Korean	Korean	99%	Buddhist and	72%
English	Other	1%	Confucianism	
			Christian	28%

Predominant Sick Care Practices: Biomedical; holistic; traditional. The body is thought to be the property of ancestors; the individual has an obligation to take care of the body. Acupuncture, herbal medicines, moxibustion, and cupping are treatments that are used often. Western and traditional treatments may be sought.

Health Care Beliefs: Active involvement; health promotion important. Mental illness is feared, is thought to be inherited, and is manifested as somatic complaints. The cause of illness is related to disturbance of the body's vital energies; symptoms may be based on psychosocial determinants. Improvement is evaluated in terms of functional ability. Belief that illness needs to be drawn out of the body is practiced through coin rubbing. A heated coin or one smeared with oil is vigorously rubbed over the body, producing red welts.

Ethnic/Race Specific or Endemic Diseases: RISK: Japanese encephalitis.

Health Team Relationships: Physicians and nurses are viewed as authority figures, treated with great respect, and not disagreed with. The response "no" might upset another person's peace of mind or mood; therefore "yes" is often the answer given, regardless of the truth.

Families' Role in Hospital Care: The family performs personal care.

Dominance Patterns: Father-son relationships are more highly regarded than are husband-wife relationships. The eldest son inherits the patriarchal position. The father makes decisions for all family members, including decisions involving health and medical care. Women have no legal rights to their children; children belong to the husband's family. Status as an elder and retirement are earned at age 60.

Eye Contact Practices: Status determines whether direct eye contact is avoided or maintained for a brief time. When looking away, the eyes are turned to the side; they are not turned up or down.

Touch Practices: Physical touching is considered an affront, particularly with the elderly. Touching among good friends of the same sex is acceptable. Physical contact between members of the opposite sex is not proper.

Time Perceptions: Punctuality is flexible; a 30-minute leeway for keeping appointments is acceptable. Rushing to be on time is considered undignified.

Pain Reactions: People tend toward stoicism. It is proper to display no facial expression.

Birth Rites: The father is not present during birth. Immediately after birth, bowls of clear water and rice may be placed in the delivery room to give thanks to the spirit who guards childbirth. Mothers avoid exposure to cold, including air conditioning, may wish to eat warm foods only, and will take no iced drinks. A son's birth is celebrated but not a daughter's.

Death Rites: Buddhist influence accepts death as birth into another life. Family members are summoned to observe the dying person's last breath and may respond with loud wailing and displays of intense emotion.

Food Practices and Intolerances: Lactose intolerance is common. Rice is a basic food; fruit is dessert. Many meals include kimchee, which is a pickled cabbage. Breakfast is the principal meal of the day.

Child Rearing Practices: Infants are not allowed to cry for long and are breastfed (on demand) until they are approximately 2 years old. Children may sleep with parents until age 4. The mother cares for the child in a permissive, affectionate atmosphere until age 7; then the father takes over supervision and tends to be more demanding, not hugging, caressing, or kissing the child. Children are expected to be humble and obedient.

National Childhood Immunizations: DPT at 2 months, 4 months, 6 months; DPT booster at 18 months; DT at 6 years; polio at 2 months, 4 months, 6 months, and 6 years; BCG at birth; measles at 15 months.

Other Characteristics: The Korean has three names: the family name is written first, the generational name second, and the given name last. The given name is used only by family and intimate friends. A woman does not change her name when she marries.

Food or drink, when first offered, will be refused out of politeness, no matter how much it is desired. The offer must be repeated. Bowel and urine elimination is done by squatting over a receptacle on the floor. Toilets with seats may be a safety hazard to people who are unfamiliar with them. Bedpans may be preferred on the floor.

BIBLIOGRAPHY

Brigham Young University Language Research Center: *Building bridges of understanding: Koreans,* Provo, Utah, 1976, Brigham Young University Press.

Choi EC: Unique aspects of Korean-American mothers, *JOGNN* 15(5):394, 1986.

Galanti GA: *Caring for patients from different cultures,* Philadelphia, 1991, University of Pennsylvania Press.

Inglis M, Gudykunst WB: Institutional completeness and communication acculturation: a comparison of Korean immigrants in Chicago and Hartford, *J Intercult Relations* 6:251, 1982.

Langer C: Contributor.

Merchant JJ: Korean interpersonal patterns: implications for Korean/American intercultural communication, Term paper, Southern Oregon State College, Ashland, Oregon, n.d.

National Association for Foreign Student Affairs: *The Republic of Korea: an educational exchange profile,* Washington, DC, 1988, The Association.

Pang KY: The practice of traditional Korean medicine in Washington, D.C., *Soc Sci Med* 28(8):875, 1989.

Park JH: Nursing administration in Korea, *Nurs Admin Q* 16(2):78, 1992.

◆ KUWAIT

MAP PAGE (262)

Location: Located on the northwest shore of the Persian Gulf, Kuwait is flat with a wide temperature range and high humidity. Most people live in cities and, to escape summer heat and humidity, are extensive travelers.

Major Languages	Ethnic Groups		Major Religions	
Arabic	Kuwaiti	39%	Sunni Muslim	45%
English	Other Arab	39%	Shi'a Muslim	30%
	South Asian	9%	Other Muslim	10%
	Iranian	4%	Christian and	
	Other	9%	Other	15%

Predominant Sick Care Practices: Biomedical; magico-religious. Belief in the evil eye exists.

Health Care Beliefs: Active involvement; health promotion is important. Intrusive procedures, such as injections and intravenous fluids, are perceived as more effective. Males tend to view illness as the inability to function; females define illness in terms of signs, symptoms, and pain. Pharmacists and nurses have the right to prescribe drugs; self-medication is practiced.

Health Team Relationships: Patients shop around continually for the ideal physician with a common ethnic background. Health history questions relating to personal or family health, business, or social status may not be answered. Medicine is male dominated; nursing is a low-esteem women's job that is marked by compliance and by following physicians' orders.

Families' Role in Hospital Care: Family and friends expect to be with the patient as much as possible and are demanding with health care personnel to ensure that the patient receives care and attention.

Dominance Patterns: By law, men and women are not equal. Passive-aggressive behaviors, rather than confrontational behaviors, are used (especially by women) to solve problems.

Eye Contact Practices: Conversations occur with approximately 2 feet separating the participants. Closeness permits evaluation of pupil responses. Pupils dilate with interest and contract with dislike.

Touch Practices: Touching is limited to members of the same sex; it is important in communication between men.

Pain Reactions: Pain relief is expected immediately and may be persistently requested. The belief in conserving energy for recovery is in conflict with therapies that require exertion. Pain is expressed privately or only with close relatives and friends. However, pain is expressed during labor and delivery.

Death Rites: Hope is valued. God is believed to know the true prognosis; therefore death or a bad prognosis is discussed with extreme reluctance. Muslim belief forbids organ donations or transplants. Muslim physicians may recommend transfusions to save lives. Autopsy is uncommon because the deceased must be buried intact. For

Muslim burial the body is wrapped in special pieces of cloth and buried without a coffin in the ground. Cremation is not permitted.

Food Practices and Intolerances: Pork, carrion, and blood are forbidden to Muslims. Food tends to be spicy. Ramadan fasting is practiced with exemptions for the sick and children.

Infant Feeding Practices: Breastfeeding is practiced by 50% of the mothers and has a duration of 16 months.

Child Rearing Practices: Public denigration of children is preferred over praise for fear of the evil eye.

National Childhood Immunizations: OPV at birth; OPV-1 at 3 months, OPV-2 at 4 months, OPV-3 at 5 months, OPV-4 at 6 months; OPV booster between 15 and 24 months. More than 90% of children are immunized.

Other Characteristics: Hope, optimism, and the positive advantages of treatment should be stressed.

BIBLIOGRAPHY

Dalayon A: Nursing in Kuwait: problems and prospects, *Nurs Manage* 21(9):129, 1990.

Green J: Death with dignity: Islam, *Nurs Times* 85(5):56, 1989.

Hall ET: Learning the Arabs' silent language, *Psychol Today* August:45, 1979.

Hathout MM: Comment on ethical crises and cultural differences, *West J Med* 139(3):380, 1983.

Meleis AI: The health care system of Kuwait: the social paradoxes, *Soc Sci Med* 13A:743, 1979.

Meleis AI: The Arab American in the health care system, *Am J Nurs* June:1180, 1981.

Meleis AI, Jonsen AR: Medicine in perspective: ethical crises and cultural differences, *West J Med* 138(6):889, 1983.

Miller K: NBC News, July 31, 1992.

Reizian A, Meleis AI: Arab-Americans' perceptions of and responses to pain, *Crit Care Nurse* 6(6):30, 1986.

Ross HM: Societal/cultural views regarding death and dying, *Top Clin Nurs* 1(1):1, 1981.

Shah NM, Shah MA: Socioeconomic and health care determinants of child survival in Kuwait, *J Biosoc Sci* 22(2):239, 1990.

Shah MA, Shah NM, Yunis MK: Allied health manpower in Kuwait: issues and answers, *J Allied Health* 19(2):117, 1990.

◆ LAOS

MAP PAGE (265)

Location: Laos is located in southeast Asia in the northeast part of the Indochinese peninsula. The land is mountainous (especially in the north) with dense forests and jungle.

Major Languages	Ethnic Groups		Major Religions	
Lao	Lao		Buddhist	85%
French	(Lao Lum)	50%	Animist	
English	Tribal Thai		and Other	15%
	(Lao Tung)	20%		
	Phoutheung			
	(Kha)	15%		
	Other	15%		

Laos has approximately 67 different ethnic groups.

Predominant Sick Care Practices: Biomedical; magico-religious; traditional. Traditional health practices are closely linked with religious traditions. The Lao believe that 32 spirits inhabit the body and govern its functioning. Herbal medicine is an important traditional practice. The medicines are classified as *cool,* while most western medicines are considered *hot.* Traditionally illness is handled with self-care and self-medication.

Health Care Beliefs: Acute sick care only. Unhealthy air currents or *bad winds* are thought to cause illness. Pinching or scratching the area and producing marks or red lines lets the *bad winds* out of the body and restores health. Wrist strings around the neck, ankles, or waist prevent soul loss, which is thought to cause illness.

Ethnic/Race Specific or Endemic Diseases: ENDEMIC: Chloroquine-resistant malaria. RISK: Japanese encephalitis; schistosomiasis in the southern regions; dengue fever; iodine deficiency in the mountainous regions.

Health Team Relationships: In traditional families the oldest male makes health care decisions. Physicians are thought to be authority figures and experts; therefore patients are told little about their conditions, the medicines, or the diagnostic procedures. As a result patients may be poor historians.

Families' Role in Hospital Care: Many family members may accompany the patient to the hospital and remain with the patient for the duration of the stay.

Dominance Patterns: The basic family unit often has 3 or 4 generations living together. Decision making is influenced by the astrologic and lunar calendars. Women defer to men's decisions in most matters of the outside world; however, women frequently control the home and the community economy.

Eye Contact Practices: Looking steadily into the eyes of someone who is respected is not proper.

Touch Practices: Because many believe that the head is the seat of life, it is revered, and invasive procedures are frightening. Only parents are permitted to touch the heads of their children. The female's breast is accepted dispassionately as the means of infant feeding, while the female's lower torso is extremely private. Women cover the area between the waist and knees, even in private. Females who sit with crossed legs are behaving offensively. Handshaking has gained wide acceptance among men; however, it is not acceptable among women. Touching or kissing between brother and sister is not allowed. Waving the hand with the palm up is not acceptable.

Perceptions of Time: Emphasis is not placed on the urgency of getting a task done. Punctuality is reserved for important circumstances.

Pain Reactions: Pain may be severe before relief is requested.

Birth Rites: The husband may or may not be welcomed in the delivery room. Circumcision is generally unknown. The newborn is not given compliments so that he or she will not be captured by evil spirits. Traditionally the woman must remain inside the home for 1 month after delivery. Traditional mothers may lie near or sit over a smoldering fire for several days after delivery to help dry up the womb. The newborn's age is considered to be 1 year at birth.

Death Rites: The preference is quality of life over quantity of life because of the belief in reincarnation and the expectation of less suffering in the next life. Death at home is preferred. Cremation and burial are practiced. People who die in hospitals or from accidents are not cremated but are taken directly from the hospital or scene of the accident to the temple and buried quickly. After death the body is cleaned and dressed in good clothes, and the face is washed with coconut water. White flowers and candles may be put into the deceased's hands. In some areas jewels or money (a wealthier family) and rice (a poorer family) will be put in the mouth of the deceased in the belief that these objects will help the soul encounter gods and devils.

Food Practices and Intolerances: Glutinous, sticky rice, a salad made of green papaya known as *tam mahoun,* and hot chilies are the main foods. *Lop* (raw or cooked meat pounded together with herbs and spices) is eaten at celebrations. *Lao-lao,* a form of locally prepared rice liquor, is particularly enjoyed by the men daily. Soup made of rice and water is a popular food for the sick.

Infant Feeding Practices: Newborns are not allowed to breastfeed until the mother has a full milk supply. The colostrum is considered poisonous and may give the infant diarrhea. For several days postpartum (weeks in the case of the first child) the mother will eat large amounts of salt and fat. During this time she does not eat red meats, fruits, or vegetables. Small amounts of chicken may be eaten.

Child Rearing Practices: Methods for calculating the age of an infant may vary by as much as 2 years. At approximately age 6 strict upbringing begins, independence is discouraged, and parents demand obedience. The oldest child (boy or girl) is responsible for younger siblings if the parents are dead, old, or ill. Segregation of females is common.

National Childhood Immunizations: DPT at 2 months, 3 months, and 5 months; polio at 2 months, 3 months, and

4 months; BCG at birth and between 6 and 8 years; measles between 9 and 23 months. Immunization coverage at the national level is quite low.

Other Characteristics: Because of stigma against mental illness, emotional disturbances may be manifested somatically. The family name is written first and followed by the given name. Married women officially use their husbands' last name. Given names are used almost exclusively. Family names are used only for formal occasions or on written documents.

BIBLIOGRAPHY

Galanti GA: *Caring for patients from different cultures,* Philadelphia, 1991, University of Pennsylvania Press.

Kurtz JR: Contributor.

Lawson LV: Culturally sensitive support for grieving parents, *MCN* 15:76, 1990.

Li GR: *Funeral practices,* New York, World Relief, n.d.

Muecke MA: Caring for Southeast Asian refugee patients in the USA, *Am J Public Health* 73(4):431, 1983.

Nguyen A, Bounthinh T, Mum S: *Folk medicine, folk nutrition, superstitions,* Washington, DC, 1980, Team Associates.

Schreiner D: S.E. Asian folk healing practices/child abuse? Indochinese Health Care Conference, Eugene, Ore, 1981.

Shellenberger J: Contributor.

Stewart EC, Bennett MJ: *American cultural patterns: a cross-cultural perspective,* rev ed, Yarmouth, Me, 1991, Intercultural Press.

Storti C: *The art of crossing cultures,* Yarmouth, Me, 1990, Intercultural Press.

Uland E, Smith S: Southeast Asian mental health issues. Unpublished paper, 1984.

U.S. Department of Health, Education, and Welfare Social Security Administration Office of Family Assistance SSA. *A guide to two cultures: Indochinese,* Washington, DC#77-21013, n.d.

Vandeusen J et al: Southeast Asian social and cultural customs: similarities and differences, *J Refugee Resettlement* 1:20, 1980.

◆ LEBANON

MAP PAGE (262)

Location: Located on the eastern end of the Mediterranean Sea, Lebanon has two mountain ranges running from north to south with the fertile agricultural Bekaa Valley in between.

Major Languages	Ethnic Groups		Major Religions	
Arabic	Arab	93%	Muslim	75%
French	Armenian	6%	Christian	
Armenian	Other	1%	and Other	25%
English				

Health Care Beliefs: Acute sick care only.

Ethnic/Race Specific or Endemic Diseases: RISK: Dyggve-Melchoir-Clausen syndrome.

Families' Role in Hospital Care: The patient is usually accompanied by one or more family members or close friends who expect to participate in care or at least take on a vigilant supervisory role.

Dominance Patterns: This is a male-dominated culture.

Time Perceptions: Planning ahead has the potential of defying God's will.

Pain Reactions: Immediate pain relief is expected and may be persistently requested. The belief in conserving energy for recovery is in conflict with therapies that require exertion. Pain tends to be expressed privately or only with close relatives and friends. During labor and delivery pain may be very expressive.

Birth Rites: Male children are preferred. Contraception is contrary to religious values.

Death Rites: Muslim belief forbids organ donations or transplants. Muslim physicians may recommend transfusions to save lives. Autopsy is uncommon because the deceased must be buried intact. Cremation is not permitted. For Muslim burial the body is wrapped in special pieces of cloth and buried without a coffin in the ground.

Food Practices and Intolerances: The national dish is *mansaf,* which is made of stewed lamb with cooked yogurt sauce served over rice. Pork, carrion, and blood are forbidden. Food tends to be spicy. Ramadan fasting is practiced with exemptions for the sick and for children.

National Childhood Immunizations: No data located.

Other Characteristics: Hope, optimism, and the positive advantages of treatment should be stressed.

BIBLIOGRAPHY

Boyle JS, Andrews MM: *Transcultural concepts in nursing care,* Glenview, Ill, 1989, Scott, Foresman/Little, Brown College Division.

Green J: Death with dignity: Islam, *Nurs Times* 85(5):56, 1989.

Kronfol NM, Bashshur R: Lebanon's health care policy: a case study in the evolution of a health system under stress, *J Public Health Policy* 10(3):377, 1989.

Meleis AI, Sorrell L: Arab American women and their birth experiences, *MCN* 6:171, 1981.

Reizian A, Meleis AI: Arab-Americans' perceptions of and responses to pain, *Crit Care Nurse* 6(6):30, 1986.

Ross HM: Societal/cultural views regarding death and dying, *Top Clin Nurs* 1(1):1, 1981.

Sadler C: Dealing with disaster, *Nurs Mirror* March 9:22, 1983.

◆ LESOTHO

MAP PAGE (261)

Location: Losotho (formerly Basutoland) is landlocked and almost completely surrounded by the eastern region of the Republic of South Africa. The country consists primarily of mountains and rocky tableland. The majority of the people live in rural areas and some can be reached only on horseback or by airplane.

Major Languages	Ethnic Groups		Major Religions	
English	Sotho	99%	Christian	80%
Sesotho	Other	1%	Indigenous Beliefs	20%
Zulu				
Xhosa				

Predominant Sick Care Practices: Biomedical; magico-religious; traditional.

Health Care Beliefs: Acute sick care only; health promotion important. Curative care is practiced; however, the government encourages primary health care.

Ethnic/Race Specific or Endemic Diseases: ENDEMIC: Tuberculosis in adults. **RISK:** Gastroenteritis among children; gonorrhea; measles; typhoid; schistosomiasis.

Health Team Relationships: In the rural areas the village chief is the leader and helps people make health care changes and decisions. Nursing care is done primarily by aides in hospitals.

Infant Feeding Practices: Mothers prefer to use powdered milk; therefore the breastfeeding period may be short.

National Childhood Immunizations: BCG at birth; DPT-1 at 3 months; DPT-2 at 4 months; DPT-3 at 5 months; measles at 9 months; OPV-1 at 3 months; OPV-2 at 4 months; OPV-3 at 5 months.

BIBLIOGRAPHY

Andriessen PP, van der Endt RP, Gotink MH: The village health worker project in Lesotho: an evaluation, *Trop Doct* 20(3):111, 1990.
Hollifield M et al: Anxiety and depression in a village in Lesotho, Africa, *Br J Psychiatry* 156:343, 1990.
Jones S, Makoae M, Thulo F: Health care in Lesotho, *Nurs Times* 84(41):39, 1988.
Mpeta AM: The private sector's contribution to primary health care in Lesotho, *Int Nurs Rev* 29(6):187, 1982.

◆ LIBERIA

MAP PAGE (260)

Location: Liberia is located on the Atlantic coast of southwest Africa. Much of the country is covered with dense tropical forests that experience a heavy annual rainfall.

Major Languages	Ethnic Groups		Major Religions	
English	African	95%	Traditional	70%
African Languages	Americo-		Muslim	20%
	Liberian	5%	Christian	10%

Health Care Beliefs: Acute sick care.

Ethnic/Race Specific or Endemic Diseases: ACTIVE: Cholera. ENDEMIC: Yellow fever; chloroquine-resistant malaria. RISK: Schistosomiasis.

Families' Role in Hospital Care: Tradition dictates that the family accompany the patient to the hospital and take care of cooking and laundry; however, central hospital services are the current trend.

Birth Rites: The traditional midwife is valued and active in rural Liberia.

Food Practices and Intolerances: Food shortages have been critical since the 1989 civil war began.

National Childhood Immunizations: BCG at birth; DPT-1 at 6 weeks; DPT-2 at 10 weeks; DPT-3 at 14 weeks; measles at 9 months; OPV at birth; OPV-1 at 6 weeks; OPV-2 at 10 weeks; OPV-3 at 14 weeks.

BIBLIOGRAPHY

Etzel RA: Liberian obstetrics, the birth and development of midwifery. A paper submitted in partial fulfillment of the requirements of the Student Project for Amity Among Nations, University of Minnesota, 1975.

Long N: Meals distributed in Liberia, *Front Lines* 32(5):7, 1992.

Weeks RM: A perspective on controlling vaccine-preventable diseases among children in Liberia, *Infect Control* 5(11):538, 1984.

◆ LIBYA

MAP PAGE (260)

Location: Libya is officially named the Socialist People's Libyan Arab Jamahiriya. The country is 92% desert and semidesert. Topography includes some mountains in the north and south and a narrow Mediterranean coastline along the northeast of Africa.

Major Languages	Ethnic Groups		Major Religions	
Arabic	Arab Berber	97%	Sunni Muslim	97%
Italian	Other	3%	Other	3%
English				

Ethnic/Race Specific or Endemic Diseases: ENDEMIC: Chloroquine-sensitive malaria (no risk in urban areas). RISK: Schistosomiasis; cystinuria.

Families' Role in Hospital Care: Family members or close friends accompany the patient and expect to participate in care or at least take on a vigilant supervisory role.

Dominance Patterns: Sociocultural and religious traditions strongly favor male dominance; however, attitudes are changing among educated young males.

Pain Reactions: Immediate pain relief is expected and may be persistently requested. The belief in conserving energy for recovery is in conflict with therapies that require exertion. Pain is expressed privately or only with close relatives and friends. However, during labor and delivery pain is very expressive.

Death Rites: Muslim belief forbids organ donations or transplants. Muslim physicians may recommend transfusions to save lives. Autopsy is uncommon because the deceased must be buried intact. Cremation is not permitted. For Muslim burial the body is wrapped in special pieces of cloth and buried without a coffin in the ground.

Food Practices and Intolerances: Pork, carrion, and blood are forbidden. Food tends to be spicy. Ramadan fasting is practiced with exemptions for the sick and children.

National Childhood Immunizations: OPV-1 at 3 months; OPV-2 at 4 months; OPV-3 at 5 months; BCG between 1 week and 1 month; DPT-1 at 3 months; DPT-2 at 4 months; DPT-3 at 5 months; DPT booster at 18 months; DT-1 at 6 years or at school entry; DT-2 at 13 years; measles at 9 months.

Other Characteristics: Hope, optimism, and the positive advantages of treatment should be stressed.

BIBLIOGRAPHY

Biri EW et al: Correlates of men's attitudes toward women's roles in Libya, *Int J Intercult Relations* 11(3):295, 1987.

Boyle JS, Andrews MM: *Transcultural concepts in nursing care,* Glenview, Ill, 1989, Scott, Foresman/Little, Brown College Division.

Green J: Death with dignity: Islam, *Nurs Times* 85(5):56, 1989.

Reizian A, Meleis AI: Arab-Americans' perceptions of and responses to pain, *Crit Care Nurse* 6(6):30, 1986.

Ross HM: Societal/cultural views regarding death and dying, *Top Clin Nurs* 1(1):1, 1981.

◆ LIECHTENSTEIN

MAP PAGE (258)

Location: The tiny country of Liechtenstein is located between Austria and Switzerland; the topography consists of a part of the Rhine Valley and the Alps.

Major Languages	Ethnic Groups		Major Religions	
German	Alemannic	95%	Catholic	83%
Alemannic	Italian and Other	5%	Protestant	7%
			Other	10%

BIBLIOGRAPHY
No data located.

◆ LUXEMBOURG

MAP PAGE (258)

Location: Luxembourg is located in western Europe and has heavy forests in the north and low, open plateaus in the south.

Major Languages	Ethnic Groups		Major Religions	
Luxembourgish	French-German	99%	Catholic	97%
German	Other	1%	Other	3%
French				
English				

National Childhood Immunizations: DPT at 2 to 3 months, 3 to 5 months, and 4 to 6 months; DPT or DT between 18 and 24 months; DT or TD between 5 and 6 years; TD at 15 years; OPV or IPV between 2 and 3 months, 3 and 5 months, 10 and 12 months, 18 and 24 months, 5 and 6 years, and at 15 years; MMR between 15 and 18 months.

BIBLIOGRAPHY

No data located.

◆ MADAGASCAR

MAP PAGE (261)

Location: This fourth largest island in the world is situated in the Indian Ocean across the Mozambique Channel of southeastern Africa. It contains a central plateau and low-lying coastal areas.

Major Languages	Ethnic Groups		Major Religions	
French	Malayo-		Indigenous	
Malagasy	Indonesian	98%	Beliefs	52%
	European		Christian	41%
	and Other	2%	Muslim	7%

Predominant Sick Care Practices: Biomedical; holistic; magico-religious (dominant).

Health Care Beliefs: Passive role; acute sick care only.

Ethnic/Race Specific or Endemic Diseases: ENDEMIC: Chloroquine-resistant malaria. RISK: Schistosomiasis.

Families' Role in Hospital Care: Family members attend the patient in the hospital.

Dominance Patterns: The extended family is important. Elders and ancestors are respected and honored. Ancestor worship is practiced.

Eye Contact Practices: Eye contact is avoided when confronting people in authority.

Touch Practices: Young boys and girls, as well as husbands and wives, avoid contact in public. Handshaking is the form of greeting. Parents are affectionate with their children.

Pain Reactions: Pain is shown and expressed.

Child Rearing Practices: Special rites are conducted for boys' circumcision, for Christians' baptism, and for the first haircut.

Death Rites: A second funeral is conducted with exhumation after 5 to 7 years.

Food Practices and Intolerances: Rice is the staple food.

Infant Feeding Practices: Breastfeeding is practiced for 2 years or longer.

National Childhood Immunizations: BCG at birth; DPT-1 at 3 months; DPT-2 at 4 months; DPT-3 at 5 months; DPT booster at 15 months; measles at 9 months; OPV-1 at 3 months; OPV-2 at 4 months; OPV-3 at 5 months; OPV booster at 15 months.

BIBLIOGRAPHY

Dahl Ø: Contributor.

◆ MALAWI

MAP PAGE (261)

Location: Malawi (formerly Nyasaland) is a landlocked country in southeast Africa. The north to south Rift

Valley is flanked with high plateaus and mountains. Lake Malawi in the Great Rift Valley occupies one fifth of the country.

Major Languages	Ethnic Groups		Major Religions	
English	Chewa	80%	Protestant	55%
Chichewa	Other	20%	Catholic	20%
Tombuka			Muslim	20%
			Other	5%

Predominant Sick Care Practices: Traditional. Some diseases, such as epilepsy, are thought to be best treated by traditional healers.

Health Care Beliefs: Acute sick care only; health promotion is important.

Ethnic/Race Specific or Endemic Diseases: ENDEMIC: Chloroquine-resistant malaria. RISK: Cholera; malnutrition; diarrhea; schistosomiasis. AIDS case rate is 48.3/100,000 people.

Health Team Relationships: Nurses are predominantly female and have a low status.

Dominance Patterns: Women are submissive in this patriarchial society. Grandmothers may hold a dominant family position and decide treatment of children, even if the decisions are in conflict with those of the mother. The eldest son assumes decision making when his father dies.

Birth Rites: Mothers remain ambulatory during labor. Finding the fetal head engaged in the pelvis before the beginning of labor is uncommon because of the smaller diameter of the pelvis. Unsterile household objects may be used to cut the umbilical cord, and local remedies including cow dung may be placed on the umbilical cord.

Death Rites: Open expression of grief with wailing is practiced.

Food Practices and Intolerances: Maize, cassava, and rice are staples. Men and young children receive family preference for available food.

Infant Feeding Practices: Breastfeeding is almost universal. In some areas a sweet liquid made from maize called Thobwa is given to infants.

Child Rearing Practices: The young child, who is tied to the back of the mother or to another female relative, maintains frequent close contact and at night often sleeps in the mother's bed or on the floor beside her bed. The expression of personal feelings and opinions is suppressed. Housework, obedience, and politeness are encouraged in girls. Boldness and participation in outside activities are encouraged in boys.

Other Characteristics: Almost half of Malawi's population is under 15 years of age, and females outnumber males. More than half the population has had no formal education, and approximately 90% reside in rural areas.

BIBLIOGRAPHY

Adler MW, editor: Statistics from the World Health Organization and the Centers for Disease Control, *AIDS* 6(10):1229, 1992.

French NV: Some aspects of midwifery practice in Malawi, *Midwives Chron Nurs Notes* 100(1191):98, 1987.

Macaulay C: Neonatal tetanus, *Nurs Times* Nov 13:32, 1985.

Mahat G, Phiri M: Promoting assertive behaviours in traditional societies, *Int Nurs Rev* 38(5):153, 1991.

Namate DE: Nursing in Malawi: challenges to nurses in leadership positions, *Nurs Admin Q* 16(2):24, 1992.

Pauley J: NBC News, June 22, 1992.

Speirs J: Midwifery education in Malawi, *Midwifery* 1(3):146, 1985.

Watts AE: A model for managing epilepsy in a rural community in Africa, *BMJ* 298(6676):805, 1989.

◆ MALAYSIA

MAP PAGE (265)

Location: Malaysia has two separate land masses. Western Malaysia is the southern part of the Malay Peninsula of southeast Asia. It is covered with tropical jungle, which is also a characteristic of its north to south mountain range. Eastern Malaysia includes Sabah and Sarawak on the island of Borneo.

Major Languages	Ethnic Groups		Major Religions	
Malay	Malay	59%	Muslim	58%
Chinese	Chinese	32%	Buddhist	30%
English	East Indian	8%	Hindu	8%
Tamil	Other	1%	Christian and Other	4%

Predominant Sick Care Practices: Biomedical; magico-religious; traditional. Traditional systems are firmly established along with an increase in the practice of modern medicine. Magical practices and belief in animism provide rationalizations for biomedical practices.

Ethnic/Race Specific or Endemic Diseases: RISK: Cholera; schistosomiasis. **ENDEMIC:** Chloroquine-resistant malaria, with no risk present in urban areas.

Birth Rites: During childbirth the mother's autonomy and control are not questioned. She may eat and drink whatever she wishes. Traditional beliefs include numerous birth taboos, which, if broken, are thought to affect the fetus adversely during pregnancy.

Death Rites: Muslim belief forbids organ donations or transplants. Muslim physicians may recommend transfusions to save lives. Autopsy is uncommon because the deceased must be buried intact. Cremation is not permitted. For Muslim burial the body is wrapped in special pieces of cloth and buried without a coffin in the ground.

Infant Feeding Practices: Breastfeeding and bottle feeding are practiced.

Child Rearing Practices: Male circumcision takes place between age 6 and 20. Taboos for menstruating women are quite common, and the Malay word for menstruation means *dirt.* Cleanliness is valued, and baths are taken several times a day by all age groups. Children's dislikes are generally accepted; therefore the mother finds it stressful to administer medicine to the sick child. Children sleep with the mother for the first few years, and they are toilet trained when they can communicate their needs verbally.

National Childhood Immunizations: BCG at birth and 12 years; DPT at 3 months, 4 months, and 5 months; DPT booster at 18 months and 6 years; polio at 3 months, 4 months, 5 months, 18 months, and 6 years.

Other Characteristics: In communication "I'll try" means "I will not consider it," and "Maybe" means "No commitment." A person's name is an integral part of his or her personality. Some patients may not give their names to the health care professional or permit photographs because they equate such actions with giving others power over their souls.

BIBLIOGRAPHY

Althens G: Personal communication, July 24, 1991.
Banks E: Temperament and individuality: a study of Malay children, *Am J Orthopsychiatry* 59(3):390, 1989.
Chen PC: Traditional and modern medicine in Malaysia, *Am J Chin Med* 7(3):259, 1979.
Horn BM: Cultural concepts and postpartal care, *Nurs Health Care* 2(9):516, 1981.
Laderman C: Commentary: cross-cultural perspectives on birth practices, *Birth* 15(2):86, 1988.
Lonergan S, Vansickle T: Relationship between water quality and human health: a case study of the Linggi River Basin in Malaysia, *Soc Sci Med* 33(8):937, 1991.
Ross HM: Societal/cultural views regarding death and dying, *Top Clin Nurs* 1(1):1, 1981.
Teoh JI: Taboo and Malay tradition, *Aust N Z J Psychiatry* 10(1A):105, 1976.

◆ MALDIVES

MAP PAGE (264)

Location: Formerly the Maldive Islands the country is made up of atolls and over 1000 islands. No island's area is greater than 5 square miles, and all areas are flat. The

Maldives are located in the Indian Ocean southwest of India. Inhabitants are primarily Islamic seafaring people. The Maldives are among the world's poorest countries.

Major Languages	Ethnic Groups		Major Religions	
Divehi	Sinhalese	40%	Sunni Muslim	90%
English	Dravidian	30%	Other	10%
	Arab and			
	Black	30%		

Ethnic/Race Specific or Endemic Diseases: Chloroquine-sensitive malaria.

Death Rites: Muslim belief forbids organ donations or transplants. Muslim physicians may recommend transfusions to save lives. Autopsy is uncommon because the deceased must be buried intact. Cremation is not permitted. For Muslim burial the body is wrapped in special pieces of cloth and buried without a coffin in the ground.

National Childhood Immunizations: BCG at birth and 5 years; DPT at 18 months, 19 months, and 20 months; DT booster at 5 years; TT at 15 years; measles at 9 months; OPV at 18 months, 19 months, and 20 months; OPV booster at 5 years.

BIBLIOGRAPHY

Bose R: Primary health care: experiences of the Maldives and Singapore, *Nurs J India* 76(4):83, 1985.

Ross HM: Societal/cultural views regarding death and dying, *Top Clin Nurs* 1(1):1, 1981.

◆ MALI

MAP PAGE (260)

Location: Mali was the French Sudan until 1920, and then it was called the Sudanese Republic until 1960. It is a west African landlocked country. The only fertile area is located in the south. The northern part of the country extends into the Sahara. The literacy rate is estimated at approximately 10%.

Major Languages	Ethnic Groups		Major Religions	
French	Mande	50%	Muslim	90%
Bambara	Peul	17%	Indigenous Beliefs	9%
	Voltaic	12%	Christian	1%
	Songhai	6%		
	Other	15%		

Ethnic/Race Specific or Endemic Diseases: ACTIVE: Cholera; yellow fever. **ENDEMIC:** Chloroquine-resistant malaria. **RISK:** Schistosomiasis.

Death Rites: Muslim belief forbids organ donations or transplants. Muslim physicians may recommend transfusions to save lives. Autopsy is uncommon because the deceased must be buried intact. Cremation is not permitted. For Muslim burial the body is wrapped in special pieces of cloth and buried without a coffin in the ground.

National Childhood Immunizations: BCG at birth; DPT-1 at 3 months; DPT-2 at 4 months; DPT-3 at 5 months; measles at 9 months; OPV at birth; OPV-1 at 3 months; OPV-2 at 4 months; OPV-3 at 5 months.

BIBLIOGRAPHY

Ross HM: Societal/cultural views regarding death and dying, *Top Clin Nurs* 1(1):1, 1981.

◆ MALTA

MAP PAGE (258)

Location: Malta consists of five islands in the center of the Mediterranean Sea. The islands have low hills in the interior and heavily indented coastlines.

Major Languages	Ethnic Groups		Major Religions	
Maltese	Italian	80%	Catholic	98%
English	Arab and Other	20%	Other	2%
Italian				

Birth Rites: A flower bud may be placed in the delivery room because the belief holds that when the bud opens, the birth will occur.

BIBLIOGRAPHY

Bates B, Turner AN: Imagery and symbolism in the birth practices of traditional cultures, *Birth* 12(1):29, 1985.

◆ MAURITANIA

MAP PAGE (260)

Location: This northwestern African country has approximately 350 miles (592 km) of coastline along the Atlantic. The north is arid and extends into the Sahara. The Senegal River valley in the south is fertile; however, famines have occurred in the past decade.

Major Languages	Ethnic Groups		Major Religions	
Hasaniya Arabic	Mixed Moor/		Muslim	99%
French	Black	40%	Other	1%
Toucouleur	Moor	30%		
Fula	Black	30%		
Sarakole				

Ethnic/Race Specific or Endemic Diseases: ACTIVE: Cholera. ENDEMIC: Yellow fever; chloroquine-resistant malaria. RISK: Schistosomiasis.

Death Rites: Muslim belief forbids organ donations or transplants. Muslim physicians may recommend transfusions to save lives. Autopsy is uncommon because the deceased must be buried intact. For Muslim burial the body is wrapped in special pieces of cloth and buried without a coffin in the ground. Cremation is not permitted.

National Childhood Immunizations: BCG at birth; DPT-1 at 3 months; DPT-2 at 4 months; DPT-3 at 5 months; measles at 9 months; OPV-1 at 3 months; OPV-2 at 4 months; OPV-3 at 5 months.

BIBLIOGRAPHY

Ross HM: Societal/cultural views regarding death and dying, *Top Clin Nurs* 1(1):1, 1981.

◆ MAURITIUS

MAP PAGE (261)

Location: The island nation Mauritius is located in the Indian Ocean east of Madagascar. It is a volcanic island surrounded by coral reefs. A central plateau is encircled by mountain peaks.

Major Languages	Ethnic Groups		Major Religions	
English	Indo-Mauritian	68%	Hindu	51%
Creole	Creole	27%	Christian	30%
French	Sino-Mauritian	3%	Muslim	17%
Hindi	Franco-Mauritian	2%	Other	2%
Urdu				

Ethnic/Race Specific or Endemic Diseases: RISK: Chloroquine-sensitive malaria in rural areas; schistosomiasis.

National Childhood Immunizations: BCG at birth; DPT-1 at 3 months; DPT-2 at 4 months; DPT-3 at 5 months; DT boosters at 2 years and 5 years; measles at 9 months; tetanus toxoid at 12 years; OPV-1 at 3 months; OPV-2 at 4 months; OPV-3 at 5 months; OPV booster at 2 years.

BIBLIOGRAPHY

No data located.

◆ MEXICO

MAP PAGE (256)

Location: Located between the United States and Central America, central Mexico is a high plateau with mountain chains on the east and west and oceanfront lowlands.

Major Languages	Ethnic Groups		Major Religions	
Spanish	Mestizo	60%	Catholic	97%
	Native		Protestant	
	American	30%	and Other	3%
	White	9%		
	Other	1%		

Predominant Sick Care Practices: Biomedical; magico-religious; traditional. Common beliefs include *mal ojo* (evil eye), *empacho* (bolus of food stuck to stomach wall), *caida de mollera* (fallen fontanelle), *susto* (result of a traumatic emotional experience), and *mal puesto* (hex or illness imposed by another).

Health Care Beliefs: Passive role; acute sick care only. People of all socioeconomic and educational levels use biomedical and folk health systems. Health is believed to be a matter of chance or God's will. Disease conditions are influenced by hot and cold imbalances. Males are perceived as being healthier than females or children, and good health in males is part of appearing *macho.* Severity of the patient's illness may be determined, in part by pain or the appearance of blood.

Ethnic/Race Specific or Endemic Diseases: ENDEMIC: Chloroquine-sensitive malaria with no risk in urban areas. RISK: Obesity; diabetes; tuberculosis; dengue fever; higher hemoglobin and hematocrit levels.

Health Team Relationships: The practitioner is viewed as an outsider. Family interdependence takes precedence over independence, so self-care is not an important concept. Personal matters are discussed and handled within the family. The *curandero* or folkhealer is a member of the nuclear or extended family network. Valued behaviors by health care practitioners are being informal and friendly, including family members in interaction, giving careful and concrete explanations, sharing experiences, taking time to listen, and inquiring about the patient's health. Health care practitioners should be the same sex as their patients.

Families' Role in Hospital Care: The male should be consulted before health care decisions are made and should be included in any counseling sessions. Culturally, a mother is not allowed the authority to give consent for her child's treatment, and family decisions supersede decisions by health care providers. Women may not give care at home if that care involves touching adult male genitalia.

Dominance Patterns: The family structure is patriarchal. The mother is in charge of running the household and decides when health care will be sought. Deference is given to elders, fathers, and grandfathers.

Eye Contact Practices: Sustained direct contact is rude, immodest, or dangerous for some. *Mal ojo* (evil eye) is the result of excessive admiration. Women and children are thought to be more susceptible to *mal ojo;* therefore children may avoid direct eye contact.

Touch Practices: Touch is used often. Touching people while complimenting them neutralizes the power of the evil eye in believers.

Perceptions of Time: The tendency is to focus on the present and to be relatively unconcerned about the future. The concept of time is a relaxed one. *Mañana* may or may not mean tomorrow.

Pain Reactions: Emotional self-restraint and stoic inhibition of strong feelings and emotional expression are seen. Expression of pain may be a self-help relief mechanism. Pain relief might be refused as a means for atonement. During labor the loud verbal repetition of "Aye, yie, yie," requires long, slow breaths, thus becoming a culturally and medically appropriate method of pain relief.

Birth Rites: Beliefs about pregnancy may include sleeping flat on the back to protect the baby, keeping active to ensure a small baby and an easy delivery, avoiding cold air, and continuing sexual intercourse to lubricate the birth canal. It is inappropriate for the husband to be with his wife during delivery; he is not expected to see his wife or child until both have been cleaned and dressed. A lying-in period of 6 weeks may be practiced. The woman rests, stays warm, avoids bathing and exercise, and eats special foods that promote warmth.

Death Rites: Small children may be shielded from dying and death rituals. Family members take turns staying around the clock with the dying person in the hospital. Grief can be expressive; for example, *el ataque* consists of hyperkinetic or seizure-type behavior patterns that serve to release emotions.

Food Practices and Intolerances: Lactose intolerance is seen. Prenatal vitamins are thought to be a *hot* food and are not to be taken during pregnancy. Dietary staples, such as rice and beans, provide complete proteins.

Infant Feeding Practices: Colostrum may be perceived as bad milk; therefore bottle feeding may be used until the breasts fill.

Child Rearing Practices: A coin is strapped firmly to the infant's navel to make the navel attractive. Most mothers are willing to wipe the coin with alcohol before putting it in place. Birth control methods other than rhythm are not popular in the Catholic population. Children are expected to respect and obey parents and their elders. Older male children may discipline younger siblings.

National Childhood Immunizations: DPT-1 between 2 and 12 months; DPT-2 between 4 and 24 months; DPT-3 between 6 and 36 months; OPV-1 between 2 and 12 months; OPV-2 between 4 and 24 months; OPV-3 between 6 and 36 months; measles at 12 months; BCG at birth.

Other Characteristics: It is believed that a high body temperature may be broken by using warm blankets and hot drinks. Except for narcotics, barbiturates, and other addictive drugs, the sale of drugs is uncontrolled, and self-medication is widely practiced. Intravenous solutions *(sueros)* are also available and may be infused at home by family members or by folk healers. The first surname is the mother's, and the second is the father's. A married woman adds "de" before the husband's surname. Human beings are measured with the palm open and held vertical to the ground at the correct height.

BIBLIOGRAPHY

Anthony-Tkach C: Care of the Mexican-American patient, *Nurs Health Care* 2(8):424, 1981.

Baca JE: Some health beliefs of the Spanish speaking, *Am J Nurs* 69(10):2172, 1969.

Boyle JS, Andrews MM: *Transcultural concepts in nursing care,* Glenview, Ill, 1989, Scott, Foresman/Little, Brown College Division.

Calatrello RL: The Hispanic concept of illness: an obstacle to effective health care management? *Behav Med* 7(11):23, 1980.

Calvillo ER, Flaskerud JH: Review of literature on culture and pain of adults with focus on Mexican-Americans, *J Transcult Nurs* 2(2):16, 1991.

Condon JC, Yousef F: *An introduction to intercultural communication,* New York, 1975, Macmillan.

Day D: A day with the dead, *Nat History* Oct:67, 1990.

Eisenbruch M: Cross-cultural aspects of bereavement. II. Ethnic and cultural variations in the development of bereavement practices, *Cult Med Psychiatry* 8(4):315, 1984.

Galanti GA: *Caring for patients from different cultures,* Philadelphia, 1991, University of Pennsylvania Press.

Giger JN, Davidhizar RE: *Transcultural nursing,* St Louis, 1991, Mosby.

Gonzalez HH: *Health beliefs of some Mexican-Americans. In Becoming aware of cultural differences in nursing,* Kansas City, 1972, American Nurses Association.

Gonzalez-Swafford MJ, Gutierrez MG: Ethno-medical beliefs and practices of Mexican-Americans, *Nurse Pract* 8(10):29, 1983.

Horn BM: Cultural concepts and postpartal care, *Nurs Health Care* 2(9):516, 1981.

Kay M: *Anthropologist of domestic care. In Barbee EL, editor: The anthropology of nurse anthropologists,* San Francisco, 1991, Council on Nursing and Anthropology.

Lawson LV: Culturally sensitive support for grieving parents, *MCN* 15:76, 1990.

Leininger MM: *Transcultural nursing: concepts, theories, and practices,* New York, 1978, John Wiley & Sons.

Lipton JA, Marbach JJ: Pain differences, similarities found, *Sci News* 118:182, 1980.

Martinelli AM: Pain and ethnicity: how people of different cultures experience pain, *AORN J* 46(2):273, 1987.

Martinez C, Martin HW: Folk diseases among urban Mexican-Americans: etiology, symptoms, and treatments, *JAMA* 196(2):147, 1966.

McKenna M: Twice in need of care: a transcultural nursing analysis of elderly Mexican-Americans, *J Transcult Nurs* 1(1):46, 1989.

Ross HM: Societal/cultural views regarding death and dying, *Top Clin Nurs* 1(1):1, 1981.

Shellenberger JM: A practice model for culturally appropriate nursing care in a primary health care setting for Mexican-American persons, doctoral dissertation, Austin, 1987, University of Texas.

Spector RE: *Cultural diversity in health and illness,* ed 3, Norwalk, Conn, 1991, Appleton & Lange.

Stewart EC, Bennett MJ: *American cultural patterns: a cross-cultural perspective,* rev ed, Yarmouth, Me, 1991, Intercultural Press.

Taylor VL, editor: *Culturgrams: the nations around us,* Provo, Utah, 1987, Brigham Young University, David M. Kennedy Center for International Studies.

◆ MONACO

MAP PAGE (258)

Location: Monaco is a tiny (0.6 square mile), hilly wedge of coastal land on the French Mediterranean.

Major Languages	Ethnic Groups		Major Religions	
French	French	47%	Catholic	95%
English	Monegasque	16%	Other	5%
Italian	Italian	16%		
Monegasque	Other	21%		

BIBLIOGRAPHY
No data located.

◆ MONGOLIA

MAP PAGE (263)

Location: Mongolia (formerly Outer Mongolia) is one of the oldest countries in the world. It is located in east central Asia. Most of the country consists of high plateaus with mountains, salt lakes, and vast grasslands. Much of the Gobi Desert is in southern Mongolia.

Major Languages	Ethnic Groups		Major Religions	
Khalkha Mongol	Mongol	90%	Tibetan Buddhist	95%
Turkish	Kazakh	4%	Muslim	4%
Russian	Chinese	2%	Other	1%
Chinese	Russian	2%		
	Other	2%		

National Childhood Immunizations: BCG between 5 and 7 days; BCG boosters at 8 years, 13 years, and 18 years; DPT at 3 months, 4 months, and 5 months; DPT boosters at 2 years, 6 years, and 11 years; measles between 9 and 13 months; OPV at 3 months, 4 months, and 5 months; OPV boosters at 2 years, 3 years, 15 years, and 18 years.

BIBLIOGRAPHY

No data located.

◆ MOROCCO

MAP PAGE (260)

Location: Morocco is located on the northwestern coast of Africa just south of Spain and across the Strait of Gibraltar. The Atlantic coast has fertile plains, while the Mediterranean coast is mountainous.

Major Languages	Ethnic Groups		Major Religions	
Arabic	Arab Berber	99%	Sunni Muslim	99%
Berber	Other	1%	Other	1%
French				

Ethnic/Race Specific or Endemic Diseases: ENDEMIC: Chloroquine-sensitive malaria (no risk in urban areas). RISK: Schistosomiasis; ataxia-telangiectasia; glycogen storage disease type III.

Families' Role in Hospital Care: Family members or close friends accompany the patient and expect to participate in care or to take on a vigilant, supervisory role.

Dominance Patterns: Men and women have contrasting social roles. The father has authority but uses it with some flexibility.

Touch Practices: It is customary for men to walk hand in hand in public.

Pain Reactions: Immediate pain relief is expected and may be persistently requested. The belief in conserving energy for recovery is in conflict with therapies that require exertion. Pain is expressed privately or only with close relatives and friends. During labor and delivery, pain is more expressive.

Death Rites: Muslim belief forbids organ donations or transplants. Muslim physicians may recommend transfusions to save lives. Autopsy is uncommon because the deceased must be buried intact. Cremation is not permitted. For Muslim burial the body is wrapped in special pieces of cloth and buried without a coffin in the ground.

Food Practices and Intolerances: Taking only the food that is being served or the food that has been served is preferable to reaching for food. Pork, carrion, and blood are forbidden. Food tends to be spicy. Ramadan fasting is practiced with exemptions for the sick and for children.

National Childhood Immunizations: No data located.

Other Characteristics: Hope, optimism, and the positive advantages of treatment should be stressed.

BIBLIOGRAPHY

Boyle JS, Andrews MM: *Transcultural concepts in nursing care,* Glenview, Ill, 1989, Scott, Foresman/Little, Brown College Division.

Green J: Death with dignity: Islam, *Nurs Times* 85(5):56, 1989.

Laaziri Z: Morocco: the big day, *World Health* Dec:27, 1984.

Murphy EJ: *Tradition and change in modern Morocco,* World Education Project, Storrs, 1974, School of Education, University of Connecticut.

Reizian A, Meleis AI: Arab-Americans' perceptions of and responses to pain, *Crit Care Nurse* 6(6):30, 1986.

Ross HM: Societal/cultural views regarding death and dying, *Top Clin Nurs* 1(1):1, 1981.

Storti C: *The art of crossing cultures,* Yarmouth, Me, 1990, Intercultural Press.

◆ MOZAMBIQUE

MAP PAGE (261)

Location: Mozambique stretches along the southeast coast of Africa. Coastal lowlands cover nearly one half of the country, and plateaus gradually rise to its western mountains. Civil war is ongoing in recent years, and the population has suffered from severe drought and famine. Crops have failed in some areas. All of these circumstances contribute to Mozambique's standing among the world's poorest countries.

Major Languages	Ethnic Groups		Major Religions	
Portuguese	Indigenous		Indigenous	
African	Groups	85%	Beliefs	60%
Languages	Other	15%	Christian	30%
			Muslim	10%

Predominant Sick Care Practices: Money for health care is currently being used for the civil war.

Health Care Beliefs: Health care is nationalized and includes a policy of primary health care.

Ethnic/Race Specific or Endemic Diseases: ENDEMIC: Chloroquine-resistant malaria. RISK: Schistosomiasis; diarrhea; hookworm; multifactorial anemia.

Birth Rites: The majority of infants are born at home. A traditional birth attendant or a relative is present. Rural infants who are born at home may be delivered onto the ground and are left untouched until the placenta is delivered. High value is placed on having a large number of children; however, couples are encouraged to space the births of their children.

Food Practices and Intolerances: Sorghum and beans are common. Oil is used sparingly in cooking.

Infant Feeding Practices: Breastfeeding is encouraged until the infant is 18 months.

National Childhood Immunizations: BCG at birth; DPT-1 at 6 weeks; DPT-2 at 10 weeks; DPT-3 at 14 weeks; measles at 9 months; OPV-1 at 6 weeks; OPV-2 at 10 weeks; OPV-3 at 14 weeks.

BIBLIOGRAPHY

Mondlane RP, deGraca AMP, Ebrahim GJ: Skin-to-skin contact as a method of body warmth for infants of low birth weight, *J Trop Pediatr* 35:321, 1989.

Pauley J: NBC News, June 22, 1992.

Powell M: Beating disease in the bush, *Nurs Times* Sep 26:19, 1984.

Raisler J: Nurse-midwifery in a developing country: maternal and child health in Mozambique, *J Nurse Midwifery* 29(6):399, 1984.

Segall M, Marzagão C: Drug revolution in Mozambique, *World Health* July, 1984.

◆ NAMIBIA

MAP PAGE (261)

Location: Namibia (formerly Southwest Africa) is bounded in part by South Africa. It is a sparsely populated part of the high plateau of southern Africa. The country is currently experiencing severe drought.

Major Languages	Ethnic Groups		Major Religions	
Afrikaans	Black	86%	Christian	60%
German	White	7%	Indigenous	
English	Mixed	7%	Beliefs	40%
African Languages				

Ethnic/Race Specific or Endemic Diseases: RISK: Chloroquine-resistant malaria; schistosomiasis.

National Childhood Immunizations: No data located.

BIBLIOGRAPHY

Pauley J: NBC News, June 22, 1992.

◆ NAURU

MAP PAGE (255)

Location: A remote island nation of only 18.2 square miles (21 square km) and 8000 people, Nauru lies just south of the equator in the western Pacific Ocean. It is ringed by dying, ashen-gray coral reefs. The water is so deep that ships cannot anchor. The nearly exhausted phosphate reserves (the island's only natural resource) have provided one of the world's highest-per-capita incomes. Strip mining has left all but one fifth of the land useless.

Major Languages	Ethnic Groups		Major Religions	
Nauruan	Nauruan	58%	Christian	95%
English	Pacific Islander	26%	Other	5%
	Chinese	8%		
	European	8%		

Ethnic/Race Specific or Endemic Diseases: ENDEMIC: Highest rate of diabetes in the world. RISK: High blood pressure; heart disease; obesity. The life expectancy rate is low. Because immigrant laborers are available to do the mining, most Nauruans follow a sedentary life-style.

Health Team Relationships: Nauruans do not respond well to aggressive, argumentative people. A friendly, nonassertive approach will most likely achieve a successful interaction.

Families' Role in Hospital Care: Most services are free. On weekdays, free consultations are available at the general hospital.

Food Practices and Intolerances: Nearly all food is imported from Australia. Water also is shipped into the island. Local fish (tainted by cadmium) are usually eaten raw, especially by children. Eating processed foods is considered a sign of affluence and contributes to obesity.

National Childhood Immunizations: No data located.

Other Characteristics: Native Nauruans are large physically. Few males survive beyond age 50. Traffic accidents cause many deaths.

BIBLIOGRAPHY

Cousteau JM: Nauru—the island planet, CBS News, July 19, 1992.
Mellor B: Paradise or hell? *Time,* August 24, 1992, pp 30-31.
Stanley D: *Micronesia handbook: guide to an American lake,* Chico, Calif, 1985, Moon.

◆ NEPAL

MAP PAGE (264)

Location: Nepal is a landlocked country in South Asia that has many mountain peaks over 20,000 feet (6096 m), including Mt. Everest, which is the earth's tallest mountain. The literacy and life expectancy rates are low. Geography and altitude influence the types of health problems and also the availability of health care.

Major Languages	Ethnic Groups		Major Religions	
Nepali	Indigenous		Hindu	90%
Newari	Groups	80%	Buddhist	9%
Tibetan	East Indian	5%	Other	1%
Other	Tibetan			
	and Other	15%		

High-altitude groups include Sherpas, Tamang, and Kirantis. Midmountain groups include Tamang, Magars, Tharus, Danuars, and Chepang. The lowland group is mostly Indian immigrants.

Predominant Sick Care Practices: Biomedical; magico-religious; traditional. Health care treatments include indigenous and western, as well as Ayurvedic medicine, which is based on identifying and maintaining a balance that is identified for a particular individual. Belief in the evil eye exists.

Ethnic/Race Specific or Endemic Diseases: ENDEMIC: Chloroquine-resistant malaria with no risk in urban areas. RISK: Cholera; Japanese encephalitis; leprosy; diarrhea; nutritional deficiencies; pneumonia; communicable diseases. Accidents are common causes of death in children.

Health Team Relationships: People are considered strangers if they are outside the patient's caste system or ethnic background. People are reluctant to call upon strangers for help. Most health service positions are held by men.

Dominance Patterns: The family unit is important. The status of women is determined by marriage.

Death Rites: Some Sherpa people express grief through singing sad songs.

Infant Feeding Practices: Breastfeeding mothers do not eat vegetables because vegetables are believed to cause diarrhea and colds. Solids and salt are begun at 6 months. Fluids may not be given to infants with diarrhea in the belief that it will cause more diarrhea.

Child Rearing Practices: Sons are preferred. Contraceptive techniques are not well known. Infants to age 6 months are massaged in oil, particularly mustard oil, and placed in the sun several times a day. The oil is absorbed by the body and adds fatty tissue. The head and face are shaped to produce high noses and wide foreheads (highly valued). This is achieved by having the infants sleep on pillows shaped with seeds. Personal feelings and opinions are rarely expressed. Discipline and obedience are encouraged.

National Childhood Immunizations: BCG at birth; DPT at 6 weeks, 10 weeks, and 14 weeks; measles at 9 months; OPV at 6 weeks, 10 weeks, and 14 weeks.

BIBLIOGRAPHY

Desjarlais RR: Poetic transformations of Yolmo "sadness," *Cult Med Psychiatry* 15(4):387, 1991.

Justice J: Can socio-cultural information improve health planning? A case study of Nepal's assistant nurse-midwife, *Soc Sci Med* 19(3):193, 1984.

Mahat G, Phiri M: Promoting assertive behaviours in traditional societies, *Int Nurs Rev* 38(5):153, 1991.

Sharma A, Ross J: Nepal: integrating traditional and modern health services in the remote area of Bashkharka, *Int J Nurs Stud* 27(4):343, 1990.

Storti C: *The art of crossing cultures,* Yarmouth, Me, 1990, Intercultural Press.
Subedi J: Modern health services and health care behavior: a survey in Kathmandu, Nepal, *J Health Soc Behav* 30(4):412, 1989.

◆ NETHERLANDS

MAP PAGE (258)

Location: The Netherlands, also known as Holland, is located on the North Sea in northwestern Europe. Most of the land is low, flat farmland. Approximately 50% is below sea level. The land is protected by dikes. The islands of the Netherlands Antilles lie in the Caribbean north of Venezuela — the largest islands are Curacao and Bonaire. The islands have complete autonomy in domestic affairs.

Major Language	Ethnic Groups		Major Religions	
Dutch	Dutch	99%	Catholic	40%
	Indonesian		Protestant	31%
	and Other	1%	Unaffiliated	
			and Other	29%

Death Rites: Active euthanasia is permitted under special circumstances.

National Childhood Immunizations: Hepatitis B for children from HBsAg-positive mothers; DPT at 3 months, 4 months, 5 months, and 11 months; injectable PV at 3 months, 4 months, 5 months, and 11 months; BCG for Mediterranean aliens at 6 months; MMR at 14 months and 9 years.

BIBLIOGRAPHY

Arrindell WA et al: Cross-national generalizability of dimensions of perceived parental rearing practices: Hungary and The Netherlands: a correction and repetition with healthy adolescents, *Psychol Rep* 65(3-2):1079, 1989.
Davis AJ, Slater PV: U.S. and Australian nurses' attitudes and beliefs about the good death, *Image* 21(1):34, 1989.
Tijhuis MA, Peters L, Foets M: An orientation toward help-seeking for emotional problems, *Soc Sci Med* 31(9):989, 1990.

◆ NEW ZEALAND

MAP PAGE (255)

Location: Located below the equator, New Zealand lies about 1200 miles (2012 km) east of Australia. It consists primarily of two islands: North Island and South Island, which are separated by Cook Strait. Though both islands are hilly and mountainous, South Island has the Southern Alps with glaciers and many high mountain peaks.

Major Languages	Ethnic Groups		Major Religions	
English	European	88%	Christian	81%
Maori	Maori	9%	Unaffiliated	
	Pacific		and Other	19%
	Islander	2%		
	Other	1%		

Predominant Sick Care Practices: Biomedical.

Ethnic/Race Specific or Endemic Diseases: Mortality from asthma is higher than expected.

Health Team Relationships: Equality is valued.

Food Practices and Intolerances: A yeast spread called Vegemite is popular.

National Childhood Immunizations: BCG at birth and for at risk groups at 13 years; measles at 12 months; rubella for girls at 11 years; DPT at 3 months and 5 months; a DT booster at 18 months; polio at 3 months, 5 months, 18 months, and 5 years.

BIBLIOGRAPHY

Clements CJ, Patel AC, Pearce NE: 1988 New Zealand national immunisation survey: methodology, *NZ Med J* 102(870):320, 1989.

Davidson GP: Grief, death and bereavement among New Zealand's Polynesian people: a community affair, *NZ Nurs J* 76(7):12, 1983.

Sears MR et al: Asthma mortality comparison between New Zealand and England, *Br Med J* 293(6558):1342, 1986.

Sears MR et al: Deaths from asthma in New Zealand, *Arch Dis Child* 61(1):6, 1986.

Sherrard I: Cross-cultural studies, *NZ Nurs J* 77(11):22, 1984.

◆ NICARAGUA

MAP PAGE (256)

Location: Nicaragua is the largest yet most sparsely populated Central American country. Its Pacific coast is volcanic and fertile. The Caribbean "Mosquito Coast" is swampy.

Major Languages	Ethnic Groups		Major Religions	
Spanish	Mestizo	69%	Catholic	95%
English	White	17%	Other	5%
Indian Languages	Black	9%		
	Native American	5%		

Health Care Beliefs: Active involvement.

Ethnic/Race Specific or Endemic Diseases: RISK: Chloroquine-sensitive malaria (minimal risk in urban areas); dengue fever.

Health Team Relationships: The Nicaraguans may be reluctant to go to a hospital.

National Childhood Immunizations: DPT-1 at 1 month; DPT-2 between 2 and 3 months; DPT-3 between 4 and 5 months; DPT booster at 1 year after DPT-3; OPV-1 at birth; OPV-2 between 1 and 2 months; OPV-3 between 3 and 4 months; OPV boosters at 1 and 5 years; measles between 9 months and 5 years; BCG at birth and 5 years.

BIBLIOGRAPHY

Radcliffe M: Nicaragua: a good example in health, *Nurs Standard* 5(38):22, 1991.

◆ NIGER

MAP PAGE (260)

Location: Located in the interior of North Africa, Niger is mostly arid desert that is part of the southern Sahara.

The country experiences periods of famine and drought. Four fifths of the land is uninhabitable desert. Larger cities may not always have electricity and running water.

Major Languages	Ethnic Groups		Major Religions	
French	Hausa	56%	Muslim	80%
Hausa	Djerma	22%	Other	20%
Djerma	Fula	8%		
	Tuareg	8%		
	Beri-Beri			
	and Other	6%		

Predominant Sick Care Practices: Holistic; traditional. Primary health care and medical practice are based on an ancient and complex traditional set of practices, including herbs, Islamic treatments of religious prayers, verses, and appeals to different spirits.

Ethnic/Race Specific or Endemic Diseases: ACTIVE: Cholera. ENDEMIC: Yellow fever; chloroquine-resistant malaria.

Health Team Relationships: Because of a belief that the mention of an illness can cause it to occur, patients may describe illness in broad and general terms, especially when children are involved.

Dominance Patterns: Polygamy is practiced. The wife is responsible for all activities related to raising children and maintaining the household.

Death Rites: Muslim belief forbids organ donations or transplants. Muslim physicians may recommend transfusions to save lives. Autopsy is uncommon because the deceased must be buried intact. Cremation is not permitted. For Muslim burial the body is wrapped in special pieces of cloth and buried without a coffin in the ground.

Infant Feeding Practices: Based on the belief that breastfeeding weakens the mother, infants are quickly weaned if the mother discovers she is pregnant again.

Child Rearing Practices: Children are sent to live with grandparents or with an older female for an unspecified period of time if the mother must work in the fields, if she becomes pregnant again, or if the children become ill. The surrogate parent assumes all responsibility (except financial) for the child.

National Childhood Immunizations: BCG at birth to 5 years; injectable triple poliomyelitis vaccine (IPV-1) at 6 weeks; IPV-2 at 10 weeks; IPV-3 at 14 weeks; DPT-1 at 6 weeks; DPT-2 at 10 weeks; DPT-3 at 14 weeks; DT booster at 16 months; measles and yellow fever at 9 months; OPV at birth; OPV-1 at 6 weeks; OPV-2 at 10 weeks; OPV-3 at 14 weeks; OPV booster at 16 months; Mobile strategy: BCG up to 59 months; IPV at 3 and 9 months; measles at 9 months.

BIBLIOGRAPHY

Chmielarczyk V: Transcultural nursing: providing culturally congruent care to the Hausa of northwest Africa, *J Transcult Nurs* 3(1):15, 1991.

Khassis U, Windsor RA: Building an infrastructure for health: a conceptual framework and application, *Hygie* 2(3):27, 1983.

Ross HM: Societal/cultural views regarding death and dying, *Top Clin Nurs* 1(1):1, 1981.

◆ NIGERIA

MAP PAGE (260)

Location: Black Africa's most populous nation is located in West Africa on the Gulf of Guinea. The southern coast has swamps, mangrove forests, tropical rain forests, a plateau of open woodland, and a semidesert region in the north.

Major Languages	Ethnic Groups		Major Religions	
English	Hausa	21%	Muslim	50%
Hausa	Yoruba	20%	Christian	40%
Yoruba	Ibo	17%	Other	10%
Ibo	Fulani	9%		
Fulani and Other	Other	33%		

Predominant Sick Care Practices: Biomedical; magico-religious; traditional. Illnesses from religious or magical causes are thought not to be best treated by western medicine. Hausa traditional healers called *surgeons* treat sprains, swellings, and other selected problems.

Ethnic/Race Specific or Endemic Diseases: RISK: Cholera; yellow fever; schistosomiasis. **ENDEMIC:** Chloroquine-resistant malaria (in urban and rural areas). Female circumcision is seen.

Dominance Patterns: Men are considered superior to women.

Pain Reactions: Many Muslim Nigerians are stoic, and they may offer their pain to Allah.

Birth Rites: Traditional birth attendants are often used for deliveries outside the hospital.

Death Rites: Muslim belief forbids organ donations or transplants. Muslim physicians may recommend transfusions to save lives. Autopsy is uncommon because the deceased must be buried intact. Cremation is not permitted. For Muslim burial the body is wrapped in special pieces of cloth and buried without a coffin in the ground.

Food Practices and Intolerances: Women who are overweight by western standards are admired.

Child Rearing Practices: Large families are common.

National Childhood Immunizations: BCG at birth; DPT-1 at 6 weeks; DPT-2 at 10 weeks; DPT-3 at 14 weeks; measles at 9 months; OPV-1 at 6 weeks; OPV-2 at 10 weeks; OPV-3 at 14 weeks.

Other Characteristics: Nigeria has the highest incidence of twins in the world. The thumbs up gesture is rude.

BIBLIOGRAPHY

Discovery Channel: A planet for the taking, March 15, 1989.

Etkin NL, Ross PJ, Muazzamu I: The indigenization of pharmaceuticals: therapeutic transitions in rural Hausaland, *Soc Sci Med* 30(8):919, 1990.

Fajemilehin RB: Factors influencing high rate of 'born-before-arrival' babies in Nigeria—a case control study in Ogbomosho, *Int J Nurs Stud* 28(1):13, 1991.

Fakeye O: Contraception with subdermal levonorgestrel implants as an alternative to surgical contraception at Llorin, Nigeria, *Int J Gynaecol Obstet* 35(4):331, 1991.

Galanti GA: *Caring for patients from different cultures,* Philadelphia, 1991, University of Pennsylvania Press.

Iiechukwu STC: Food dreams and illness among Nigerians: a pilot study, *Psychiatr J Univ Ottawa* 10(2):89, 1985.

Laoye JA: Selling health in the market place: the Araromi approach, *Int J Health Educ* 23(2):87, 1980.

Odebiyi AI: The sociocultural factors affecting health care delivery in Nigeria, *J Trop Med Hyg* 80(11):249, 1977.

Onyejiaku EE et al: Evaluation of a primary health care project in Nigeria, *Int Nurs Rev* 37(3):265, 1990.

Ross HM: Societal/cultural views regarding death and dying, *Top Clin Nurs* 1(1):1, 1981.

Stewart EC, Bennett MJ: *American cultural patterns: a cross-cultural perspective,* rev ed, Yarmouth, Me, 1991, Intercultural Press.

Westbrook MT, Nordholm LA, McGee JE: Cultural differences in reactions to patient behaviour: a comparison of Swedish and Australian health professionals, *Soc Sci Med* 19(9):939, 1984.

◆ NORWAY

MAP PAGE (258)

Location: Norway occupies the western part of the Scandinavian peninsula in northwest Europe and extends approximately 300 miles (483 km) above the Arctic Circle. More than two thirds of the country is uninhabitable because of glaciers, mountains, moors, and rivers.

Major Languages	Ethnic Groups		Major Religions	
Norwegian	Norwegian	99%	Lutheran	94%
Lapp	Lappish	1%	Other Christian	4%
Finnish			Other	2%

Predominant Sick Care Practices: Biomedical; holistic.

Health Care Beliefs: Active involvement; health promotion important. Cleanliness, rest, and taking cod liver oil are believed to promote health.

Ethnic/Race Specific or Endemic Diseases: RISK: Cholestasis-lymphedema; Krabbe disease; phenylketonuria.

Health Team Relationships: The people want to be given options and to be helped in making decisions. Politeness is practiced; however, it is subject to reciprocity. The word for "sir" does not exist in the Norwegian language, and some may feel uncomfortable if "sir" is used to address them. In communication the understatement is preferred.

Families' Role in Hospital Care: Staff provides all care in the hospital. Visiting hours are fairly liberal, and young children can visit.

Dominance Patterns: Decisions are usually not made quickly; matters are debated at length. Those in the home share decision making, caring for children, and duties.

Eye Contact Practices: Direct eye contact occurs during conversations, but the eyes may shift back and forth at times.

Touch Practices: This culture has little or no touching contact. Younger people are beginning to touch more often when greeting or when saying farewell. In familiar situations, touching may be increased.

Time Perceptions: The people are present and future oriented. A general attitude persists that if things are going okay, why worry? The people are rather punctual and may give themselves a 5- to 10-minute leeway.

Birth Rites: Prenatal care and natural childbirth are common. The father often is in the delivery room to support the mother. Circumcision is not practiced.

Death Rites: The closest family members usually are with the dying person because they believe that no one should die alone. A ceremony accompanies cremation and burial in the ground.

Food Practices and Intolerances: The main meal is at midday in rural areas. More people work in the cities, so the main meal is in the early evening. City people have a sandwich for lunch, and breakfast is a heavy meal. Potatoes with meat or meatballs and boiled fish are the food staples. Great quantities of milk are consumed. Another light meal is eaten between 8 and 10 PM.

Infant Feeding Practices: Breastfeeding is encouraged and is common.

Child Rearing Practices: Because child-rearing practices are permissive, children are allowed to participate in decision making and generally have a great deal of autonomy. Children begin school at age 7.

National Childhood Immunizations: Tetanus; pertussis; measles; polio.

Other Characteristics: Homeopathic medicine and holistic approaches with acupuncture are on the increase.

BIBLIOGRAPHY

Boyle JS, Andrews MM: *Transcultural concepts in nursing care,* Glenview, Ill, 1989, Scott, Foresman/Little, Brown College Division.

Dahl Ø: Contributor.

Geissler EM: Personal observations, Aug 15-21, 1992.

Grimsmo A, Siem H: Factors affecting primary health care utilization, *Fam Pract* 1(3):155, 1984.

Habert K, Lillebo A: Made in Norway: Norwegians as others see them. *The Sons of Norway Viking,* 96-98, 1988.

Hopp Z: *Norwegian folklore simplified,* 1991, John Grieg Produksjon A/S (Translated by Toni Ramholt).

Ro OC et al: Intervention studies among elderly people, *Scand J Prim Health Care* 5(3):163, 1987.

Spector RE: *Cultural diversity in health and illness,* ed 3, Norwalk, Conn, 1991, Appleton & Lange.

◆ OMAN

MAP PAGE (262)

Location: Oman is located on the tip of the Arabian peninsula. It has a narrow coastal plain, a wide, mostly waterless plateau, and a range of barren mountains. Oil has become the major source of income.

Major Languages	Ethnic Groups		Major Religions	
Arabic	Arab	88%	Ibadhi Muslim	75%
English	Baluchi	4%	Other Muslim	20%
Baluchi	Persian	3%	Other	5%
Urdu	East Indian	2%		
Indian	African			
Languages	and Other	3%		

Ethnic/Race Specific or Endemic Diseases: ENDEMIC: Chloroquine-sensitive malaria.

Death Rites: Muslim belief forbids organ donations or transplants. Muslim physicians may recommend transfusions to save lives. Autopsy is uncommon because the deceased must be buried intact. Cremation is not permitted. For Muslim burial the body is wrapped in special pieces of cloth and buried without a coffin in the ground.

Food Practices and Intolerances: Pork, carrion, and blood are forbidden. Food tends to be spicy. Ramadan fasting is practiced with exemptions for the sick and children.

National Childhood Immunizations: OPV at birth; OPV-1 at 3 months; OPV-2 at 5 months; OPV-3 at 7 months; OPV booster between 15 and 24 months; BCG at birth; hepatitis at birth and 7 months; measles at 9 months; DPT-1 at 3 months; DPT-2 at 5 months; DPT-3 at 7 months; DPT booster at 19 months; DT-1 at 6 years or entry into school; DT-2 at 12 years.

BIBLIOGRAPHY

Ross HM: Societal/cultural views regarding death and dying, *Top Clin Nurs* 1(1):1, 1981.

◆ PAKISTAN

MAP PAGE (264)

Location: Pakistan's Hindu Kush and Himalayan mountains contain the second highest peak in the world. There are desert lands in the east and areas of alluvial plains.

Major Languages	Ethnic Groups		Major Religions	
Urdu	Punjabi	66%	Sunni Muslim	77%
English	Sindhi	13%	Shi'a Muslim	20%
Punjabi	Pashtun	9%	Other	3%
Sindhi	Baluchi and			
Pashtu	Other	12%		
and Other				

Predominant Sick Care Practices: Allopathic and indigenous medical practitioners are used.

Health Care Beliefs: Acute sick care. Approximately one third of the population has access to safe drinking water, and approximately one sixth has access to sanitation facilities.

Ethnic/Race Specific or Endemic Diseases: ENDEMIC: Chloroquine-resistant malaria (including urban areas).

Health Team Relationships: Women may object to being examined by a male physician. Criticizing someone of higher status or rank is viewed as unacceptable. Traditionally men fill positions of authority; therefore female health care workers are under the authority of male physicians and hospital administrators. Nursing is perceived as a menial occupation, and nurses are not trained to make decisions or as change agents.

Dominance Patterns: Women are expected to be obedient to male authority; women are not encouraged to make decisions.

Eye Contact Practices: The peripheral gaze or no eye contact may be preferred during interactions.

Birth Rites: The maternal and infant mortality rates are high. Approximately one fourth of births are attended by trained health personnel.

Death Rites: Muslim belief forbids organ donations or transplants. Muslim physicians may recommend transfusions to save lives. A Holy Iman does not have to be present at death; however, a Muslim should help the patient or recite the Declaration of the Faith: "There is no God but God, and Muhammed is his Messenger." According to Islamic tradition the family members must wash the body before the funeral. Autopsy is uncommon because the deceased must be buried intact. Cremation is not permitted. For Muslim burial the body is wrapped in special pieces of cloth and buried without a coffin in the ground.

Food Practices and Intolerances: During hot weather the foods that are considered *hot* (beef, pork, potatoes, and whiskey), are avoided. *Cold* foods (chicken, fish, fruit, and beer) are avoided in the winter. Pork, carrion, and blood are forbidden to Muslims. Food tends to be spicy. Ramadan fasting is practiced with exemptions for the sick.

National Childhood Immunizations: OPV at birth; OPV-1 at 2 months; OPV-2 at 3 months; OPV-3 at 4 months; OPV boosters between 15 and 24 months and 6 and 8 years.

Other Characteristics: Mortality statistics are higher for women than men, possibly because men receive preferential treatment. Most women are not literate.

BIBLIOGRAPHY

Ahmad WI: Patients' choice of general practitioner: intolerance of patients' fluency in English and the ethnicity and sex of the doctor, *JR Coll Gen Pract* 39(321):153, 1989.

Edwards N: McMaster's link with Pakistan, *Cancer Nurse* 30, March 1989.

Galanti GA: *Caring for patients from different cultures,* Philadelphia, 1991, University of Pennsylvania Press.

Harnar R et al: Health and nursing services in Pakistan: problems and challenges for nurse leaders, *Nurs Admin Q* 16(2):52, 1992.

Irujo S: *An introduction to intercultural differences and similarities in nonverbal communication.* In Wurzel JS, editor: *Toward multiculturalism,* Yarmouth, Me, 1988, Intercultural Press.

Lally MM: Last rites and funeral customs of minority groups, *Midwife Health Visit Community Nurse* 14(7):224, 1978.

Ross HM: Societal/cultural views regarding death and dying, *Top Clin Nurs* 1(1):1, 1981.

Schmidt RL: Women and health care in rural Pakistan, *Soc Sci Med* 17(7):419, 1983.

Weisfeld GE: Sociobiological patterns of Arab culture, *Ethnology Sociobiol* 11:23, 1990.

◆ PANAMA

MAP PAGE (256)

Location: Panama is the southernmost of the Central American nations. Eastern Panama is tropical rain forest, with moderate-sized hills in the interior and volcanic mountains in the west.

Major Languages	Ethnic Groups		Major Religions	
Spanish	Mestizo	70%	Catholic	93%
English	Native American	14%	Protestant	7%
	White and Other	16%		

Ethnic/Race Specific or Endemic Diseases: ENDEMIC: Yellow fever. RISK: Chloroquine-sensitive and chloroquine-resistant malaria.

National Childhood Immunizations: DPT-1 at 2 months; DPT-2 at 4 months; DPT-3 at 6 months; DPT boosters at 18 months and at 5 years; OPV at birth; OPV-1 at 2 months; OPV-2 at 4 months; OPV-3 at 6 months; OPV boosters at 18 months and at 5 years; measles at 9 months, 15 months, and 6 years; BCG at birth, 6 years, and 12 years.

Other Characteristics: Having body fat is considered healthy in women and a sign of fertility.

BIBLIOGRAPHY

Galanti GA: *Caring for patients from different cultures,* Philadelphia, 1991, University of Pennsylvania Press.

◆ PAPUA NEW GUINEA

MAP PAGE (255)

Location: Papua is located one degree below the equator on the eastern half of the island of New Guinea. The country's center is thickly forested with dense jungle and relatively unexplored mountains. The climate is temperate. The coastal lowlands are tropical. Over time the inhabitants were isolated by the topography, and an extremely large number of diverse tribes evolved. Over 700 different languages and dialects are spoken. Because of the vast number of languages and dialects, Pidgin English or Melanesian pidgin is the universal language used.

Major Languages	Ethnic Groups		Major Religions	
Pidgin English	Papua/		Christian	60%
Motu	Melanesian	95%	Indigenous	
English	Other	5%	Beliefs	30%
Other			Other	10%

Predominant Sick Care Practices: Biomedical; magico-religious; traditional. It is believed that evil spirits inhabit some jungle and forest areas.

Health Care Beliefs: Acute sick care; health promotion is important.

Ethnic/Race Specific or Endemic Diseases: ENDEMIC: Chloroquine-resistant malaria in the lowlands and coastal areas. RISK: Burkitt's lymphoma in children; pigbel (enteritis necroticans) in the highlands; anemia in all age groups; tuberculosis in children.

Health Team Relationships: Government aid posts are staffed by people trained in first aid and basic hygiene and are scattered throughout the country.

Families' Role in Hospital Care: Almost all parents actively participate in giving care to their children in the hospital.

Dominance Patterns: Obtaining the husband's approval for initiation of contraceptives is important. Male dominance and individuality are important to some. Polygamy is practiced. In rural areas women are responsible for food, children, and tending animals. Girls may be married by the age of 14.

Birth Rites: Approximately two thirds of women receive some antenatal care. The majority of births are unsupervised.

Death Rites: Women in some cultural groups are expected to express grief; however, men are not.

Food Practices and Intolerances: Sweet potatoes are eaten in the highlands, and sago palm (almost pure starch) is eaten in the lowlands.

Infant Feeding Practices: To encourage breastfeeding, prescriptions are required to obtain infant feeding bottles.

National Childhood Immunizations: DPT at 2 months, 4 months, and 6 months; polio at 2 months, 4 months, and 6 months; BCG at birth; measles at 6 months; pigbel vaccine is provided in the highlands.

BIBLIOGRAPHY

Avue B, Freeman P: Some factors affecting acceptance of family planning in Manus, *PNG Med J* 34(4):270, 1991.

Biddulph J: Child health in Papua New Guinea: a 30 year personal perspective, *Med J Aust* 154(7):439, 1991.

Discovery Channel: Jungle Trek, Sept 9, 1992.

Frankel S, Smith D: Conjugal bereavement amongst the Huli people of Papua New Guinea, *Br J Psychiatry* 141:302, 1982.

Leininger MM: Transcultural care diversity and universality: a theory of nursing, *Nurs Health Care* 6(4):209, 1985.

Marshall LB, Lakin JA: Antenatal health care policy, services and clients in urban Papua New Guinea, *Int J Nurs Stud* 21(1):19, 1984.

◆ PARAGUAY

MAP PAGE (258)

Location: A landlocked country located in southcentral South America, eastern Paraguay has grassy lands and fertile plains, while western Paraguay is covered with marshes, lagoons, dense forests, and jungles. Because Paraguay is below the equator, the seasons are reversed.

Major Languages	Ethnic Groups		Major Religions	
Spanish	Mestizo	95%	Catholic	90%
Guarani	Other	5%	Other	10%

Ethnic/Race Specific or Endemic Diseases: Chloroquine-sensitive malaria.

Touch Practices: The conversation space is close for talking with friends. Men may embrace when greeting after long absences. Close friends of both sexes may walk arm-in-arm.

National Childhood Immunizations: DPT-1 at 1 month; DPT-2 at 3 months; DPT-3 at 5 months; OPV-1 at 1 month; OPV-2 at 3 months; OPV-3 at 5 months; measles at 9 months; BCG at birth, 7 years, and 12 years.

BIBLIOGRAPHY

Tyler L: *Culturgrams: the nations around us,* vol 1, Provo, Utah, 1987, David M. Kennedy Center for International Studies, Brigham Young University.

◆ PERU

MAP PAGE (258)

Location: This western South American country along the Pacific Ocean is divided by the Andes Mountains into three zones: the arid coastline, the mountains, with peaks over 20,000 feet (6,096 m) and deep valleys, and the heavily forested eastern mountain slopes.

Major Languages	Ethnic Groups		Major Religions	
Spanish	Native American	45%	Catholic	95%
Quechua	Mestizo	37%	Other	5%
Aymara	White	15%		
	Other	3%		

Ethnic/Race Specific or Endemic Diseases: ACTIVE: Yellow fever. **RISK:** Chloroquine-sensitive and chloroquine-resistant malaria (not in urban areas); cholera.

Dominance Patterns: Males dominate.

National Childhood Immunizations: DPT-1 at 2 months; DPT-2 at 3 months; DPT-3 at 4 months; OPV at birth; OPV-1 at 2 months; OPV-2 at 3 months; OPV-3 at 4 months; measles at 9 months; BCG at birth and at 6 years.

BIBLIOGRAPHY

Bonner R: A reporter at large: Peru's war, *New Yorker* Jan:31, 1988.
Penny M, Paredes P: A competition to promote weaning foods, *World Health Forum* 10(1):99, 1989.
World Monitor TV: April 11, 1991.

◆ PHILIPPINES

MAP PAGE (265)

Location: An archipelago off the southeast coast of Asia, the Philippines consists of about 7000 volcanic islands. The larger islands are crossed with mountain ranges. More than half of the 60 million people live in extreme poverty.

Major Languages	Ethnic Groups		Major Religions	
Pilipino (Tagalog)	Christian		Catholic	83%
English	Malay	92%	Protestant	9%
Other	Muslim		Muslim	5%
	Malay	4%	Buddhist	
	Chinese	2%	and Other	3%
	Other	2%		

Predominant Sick Care Practices: Biomedical; magico-religious. A combination of home remedies, professional providers, and traditional healers is consulted. Fatalism accompanies beliefs that ghosts and spirits control life and death. Usurping the powers of the gods is believed to have a cause and effect relationship to subsequent bad happenings.

Health Care Beliefs: Acute sick care; health promotion is important. Mental illness is highly stigmatized in the Filipino culture. It is believed that the evil eye can be cast upon someone through the eyes or the mouth.

Ethnic/Race Specific or Endemic Diseases: ENDEMIC: Chloroquine-sensitive and chloroquine-resistant malaria (not in urban areas). RISK: Japanese encephalitis; schistosomiasis.

Health Team Relationships: Authority is respected, and it is believed that the professional's time is valuable; therefore the problem must be serious, or it is left unmentioned. Nurses may carry out a physician's order rather than question it. Rather than give a "no" answer, the patient may remain silent or respond with a hesitant "yes." Group decisions are often made by an influential group member. An intermediary may be used for confrontational situations.

Families' Role in Hospital Care: A child may feel an obligation to the parent who is ill and spend hours giving care. The family may desire to give physical care.

Dominance Patterns: The self is perceived in the context of the family. Protection against outsiders, reciprocity of obligation, dependency, and harmony are group values. Dependence strengthens relationships among people.

Eye Contact Practices: Some may fear eye contact; however, if it is established, it is important to return and to maintain eye contact.

Touch Practices: In some parts of the country it is believed that the evil eye may be neutralized on a child by putting a bit of saliva on the finger and making the sign of the cross on a child's forehead when giving a compliment. Touch is stressed.

Time Perceptions: Time generally moves ahead slowly. Life is lived from day to day.

Pain Reactions: People may appear stoic, believing that pain is the will of God and that God will give them the strength to bear it.

Birth Rites: It is believed that daily bathing and shampooing during pregnancy will produce a clean baby and that sexual intercourse may cause harm to the woman and the infant. Some type of symbolic unlocking or opening act during labor using keys or flowers may be practiced. A traditional postpartum lying-in period of 10 days prohibits bathing or showering. A special bath after 2 weeks removes the debris of pregnancy believed to be found in perspiration. Regardless of room temperature the new mother may wear warm clothing and keep covered with blankets.

Death Rites: The patient should be protected from knowing about a poor prognosis because it will only add to his or her suffering. After death emotional grief responses may occur.

Food Practices and Intolerances: Rice is preferred with every meal.

Infant Feeding Practices: The percentage of population involved in and the duration of breastfeeding have declined in the past two decades.

National Childhood Immunizations: BCG at 3 months and at school entry; measles between 9 and 14 months; DPT at 3 months and at 9 months; polio at 3 months, 6 months, and 9 months. Only 25% of the children are immunized against tuberculosis, diphtheria, pertussis, tetanus, polio, and measles.

Other Characteristics: The Filipino gesture that invites others to approach uses the whole hand, with palm in and fingers up. A *Quackdoctor* is a completely acceptable folk health practitioner. Premature birth weight is suggested at 2200 grams. An invitation must be extended more than once and must be reluctantly accepted. The value of shared rather than private possessions or property is practiced.

BIBLIOGRAPHY

Aguilar DD: The social construction of the Filipino woman, *Int J Intercult Relations* 13:527, 1989.

Althen GL, Jaime J: Assumptions and values in Philippine, American and other cultures, class materials, Summer Institute of Intercultural Communication, Portland, Ore, 1991.

Bates B, Turner AN: Imagery and symbolism in the birth practices of traditional cultures, *Birth* 12(1):29, 1985.

Boyle JS, Andrews MM: *Transcultural concepts in nursing care,* Glenview Ill, 1989, Scott, Foresman/Little, Brown College Division.

Condon JC, Yousef F: *An introduction to intercultural communication,* New York, 1975, Macmillan.

Davis CF: Culturally responsive nursing management in an international health care setting. In Brown BJ, editor: On the scene, *Nurs Admin Q* 16(2):36, 1992.

Galanti GA: *Caring for patients from different cultures,* Philadelphia, 1991, University of Pennsylvania Press.

Giger JN, Davidhizar RE: *Transcultural nursing,* St Louis, 1991, Mosby.

Horn BM: Cultural concepts and postpartal care, *Nurs Health Care* 2(9):516, 1981.

Lieban RW: Urban Philippine healers and their contrasting clienteles, *Cult Med Psychiatry* 5(3):217, 1981.

Luyas G: How Filipino mothers care for their young children, *UT Nurse* 5(1):7, 1991.

Marcos I: The Today Show, NBC, Oct 9, 1991.

Overfield T: *Biologic variation in health and illness,* Menlo Park, Calif, 1985, Addison-Wesley.

Prosser MH: *The cultural dialogue,* Washington, DC, 1985, SIETAR.

Ross HM: Societal/cultural views regarding death and dying, *Top Clin Nurs* 1(1):1, 1981.

Samovar LA, Porter RE: *Intercultural communication: a reader,* Belmont, Calif, 1985, Wadsworth.

Spector RE: *Cultural diversity in health and illness,* ed 3, Norwalk, Conn, 1991, Appleton & Lange.

Utley G: NBC News: Nov 3, 1991.

Williamson NE: Breastfeeding trends and the breastfeeding promotion program in the Philippines, *Int J Gynaecol Obstet Suppl 1,* 30(1)35, 1990.

◆ POLAND

MAP PAGE (258)

Location: Other than the Carpathia mountains along the south, this northcentral European country is primarily rich agricultural lowland plains.

Major Language	Ethnic Groups		Major Religions	
Polish	Polish	99%	Catholic	95%
	Ukranian		Uniate	
	and Other	1%	and other	5%

Predominant Sick Care Practices: Biomedical; magico-religious; folk. Older generations believe in the evil eye *(Szatan)* and in prayer and wearing religious medals and scapulars to help protect them against illness. Folk healers and miracle workers are also sought.

Health Care Beliefs: Passive role; acute sick care.

Ethnic/Race Specific or Endemic Diseases: RISK: Phenylketonuria.

Families' Role in Hospital Care: Parents may wish to be involved in caring for their hospitalized child.

Dominance Patterns: Traditionally the man of the family is the chief disciplinarian and decision maker; however, Poland's legal Family Code stresses equality between husband and wife. Sons are preferred over daughters.

Eye Contact Practices: Direct eye contact is made.

Touch Practices: Hugging and kissing on the cheek is acceptable between sexes.

Pain Reactions: Tolerance of pain is valued. Pain may be expressed by facial grimaces or by crying out.

Birth Rites: Among the more traditional people, preparations for birth may be made in secret to avoid evil spells. Circumcision is not universal. Recent political and economic events have influenced an increase in premature deliveries and in low-birth-weight newborns.

Death Rites: The body is not embalmed. It is placed in the home for the wake. Church services and burial in the ground follow. Feelings of grief may be verbally expressive.

Food Practices and Intolerances: The diet tends to be higher in starch and fat. Potatoes, rye, and wheat products are staples.

Child Rearing Practices: A wide variety of family planning methods are used, and abortion is an option. Strict discipline, respect for elders, and development of strength, individualism, and self-sufficiency are important. The grandmother has a valued position in child rearing.

National Childhood Immunizations: BCG at 3 to 15 days and repeated between 11 and 12 months, 6 years, 12 years, and 18 years for nonreactors; DPT at 3 months, between 4 and 5 months, 6 months, and between 19 and 24 months; DT at 7 and 14 years; OPV at 3 months, between 4 and 5 months, 6 months, between 19 and 24 months, 7 years, and 11 years; measles between 13 and 15 months; rubella for girls at 13 years.

BIBLIOGRAPHY

Boyle JS, Andrews MM: *Transcultural concepts in nursing care,* Glenview, Ill, 1989, Scott, Foresman/Little, Brown College Division.
Chilicki CR: Contributor.
Frackiewicz L: The importance of social policy in the protection of people's health in Poland, *Acta Med Leg Soc (Liege)* 36(2):35, 1986.
Lagowska U: System of nursing care in Poland, *Int Nurs Rev* 34(5):131, 1987.
Lenartowicz H: Polish nursing in action, *Nurs Admin Q* 16(2):64, 1992.
Ostrowska A: Elements of the health culture of Polish society, *Soc Sci Med* 17(10):631, 1983.
Spector RE: *Cultural diversity in health and illness,* ed 3, Norwalk, Conn, 1991, Appleton & Lange.

◆ PORTUGAL

MAP PAGE (258)

Location: Portugal is located at the extreme southwest edge of Europe on the Iberian Peninsula. It is crossed by many small rivers; the three largest arise in Spain and flow into the Atlantic. North of the Tajus River it is mountainous, cool, and rainy, while in the south dry plains and warm climate prevail. The nine islands of the Azores provide an important link in the air route across the Atlantic ocean.

Major Language	Ethnic Groups		Major Religions	
Portuguese	Portuguese	99%	Catholic	97%
	African		Protestant	1%
	and Other	1%	Other	2%

Ethnic/Race Specific or Endemic Diseases: Joseph disease.

Death Rites: The traditional widow is expected to remain unmarried and to wear black clothing for the rest of her life. She visits the grave frequently and has a picture of the deceased spouse evident in the home.

National Childhood Immunizations: BCG at birth; DPT at 3 months, 5 months, 7 months, between 18 and 24 months, and between 5 and 6 years; tetanus between 10 and 12 years; OPV at 3 months, 5 months, 7 months, between 18 and 24 months, 5 and 6 years, and 10 and 12 years; MMR after 12 months; rubella for girls between 11 and 13 years.

BIBLIOGRAPHY

Boyle JS, Andrews MM: *Transcultural concepts in nursing care,* Glenview, Ill, 1989, Scott, Foresman/Little, Brown College Division.

Eisenbruch M: Cross-cultural aspects of bereavement. II. Ethnic and cultural variations in the development of bereavement practices, *Cult Med Psychiatry* 8(4):315, 1984.

Patient education in selected countries, *J Hum Hypertens* Feb:107, 1990.

◆ QATAR

MAP PAGE (262)

Location: This Islamic republic occupies a small peninsula in the Persian Gulf. The barren, stony land is low lying; the highest point is 344 feet (105 m) above sea level. Most of its people live in the urban capital area, and the nomadic Bedouins are being encouraged to live there also.

Major Languages	Ethnic Groups		Major Religions	
Arabic	Arab	40%	Muslim	95%
English	Pakistani	18%	Other	5%
	East Indian	18%		
	Iranian	10%		
	Other	14%		

Death Rites: Muslim belief forbids organ donations or transplants. Muslim physicians may recommend transfusions to save lives. Autopsy is uncommon because the deceased must be buried intact. Cremation is not permitted. For Muslim burial the body is wrapped in special pieces of cloth and buried without a coffin in the ground.

Food Practices and Intolerances: Pork, carrion, and blood are forbidden. Food tends to be spicy. Ramadan fasting is practiced with exemptions for the sick and for children.

National Childhood Immunizations: OPV-1 at 2 months; OPV-2 at 3 months; OPV-3 at 6 months; OPV boosters between 15 and 24 months and 6 and 8 years.

BIBLIOGRAPHY

Green J: Death with dignity: Islam, *Nurs Times* 85(5):56, 1989.
Ross HM: Societal/cultural views regarding death and dying, *Top Clin Nurs* 1(1):1, 1981.

◆ ROMANIA

MAP PAGE (258)

Location: This eastern European republic opens onto the Black Sea. The highest peak of the Carpathian mountains and Transylvanian Alps is 8346 feet (2544 m) with a plateau and plains between them. Warm summers and cold, snowy winters are characteristic.

Major Languages	Ethnic Groups		Major Religions	
Romanian	Romanian	89%	Romanian	
Hungarian	Hungarian	8%	Orthodox	80%
German	German	2%	Catholic	6%
	Other	1%	Other	14%

Predominant Sick Care Practices: Biomedical; magico-religious. Superstitions and rituals are incorporated into daily life.

Health Care Beliefs: Acute sick care only.

Ethnic/Race Specific or Endemic Diseases: RISK: Industrial pollution influences health. Respiratory illnesses and cancer statistics are rising, and approximately 80% of the water supply is not potable.

Health Team Relationships: Physicians are the only health care professionals. Nursing schools were closed in 1978, and women are trained in industrial occupations.

Families' Role in Hospital Care: Patient care is at a minimum. The majority of hospitals accommodate two patients per bed. Medical equipment is not readily available, or it is kept for personal use or sold on the black market.

Dominance Patterns: The traditional pattern is patriarchal and is based on male decision making in the public domain. Although men agree that physical abuse is unacceptable, female abuse is a societal male coping mechanism. Females have authority over domestic affairs. Couples often live with the husband's parents, and the mother-in-law manages domestic affairs.

Time Perceptions: Time schedules are followed more precisely in urban areas than they are in rural areas.

Death Rites: Romanians believe in an afterlife.

National Childhood Immunizations: BCG between 4 and 60 days, between 6 and 7 years, at 13 years, and between 17 and 20 years; DPT at 3 months, 4 months, 5 months, 11 months, and 29 months; DT at 14 years; two doses of OPV at 6 week intervals between 45 days and 8 months; OPV between 10 and 15 months and at 9 years; measles between 9 and 14 months.

Other Characteristics: Abortion and contraceptives are legal. Only since the 1989 revolution has the government acknowledged the existence of AIDS. Children are often left at orphanages.

BIBLIOGRAPHY

Awlasewicz A: Contributor.

Betrothal and marriage, *Life* 14(2):54, 1991.

Buchanan J: Ceausescu's legacy, *Nurs Times* 86(7):16, 1990.

Campbell NN, Harbonne DJ, Norwich R: Medicine in Romania, *Br Med J* 300(6726):699, 1990.

Cassidy MD: Romania: haemodialysis, handicap and a sense of humor, *Lancet* 337(8737):353, 1991.

Cole JW, Nydon JA: Class, gender and fertility, *East European Q* 23(4):469, 1989.

Death and remembrance, *Life* 14(2):72, 1991.

Dickman S: AIDS in children adds to Romania's troubles, *Nature* 343:579, 1990.

Ember L: Pollution chokes East-bloc nations, *Chem Engin News* 68(16):7, 1990.

Freedman DC: Gender identity and dance style, *East Eur Q* 23(4):419, 1990.

Hale J: *Customs and folklore.* In *The land and people of Romania,* New York, 1972, Lippincott.

Lass A: The wedding of the dead, *Am Anthropol* 92(3):784, 1990.

Life after Ceausescu, *Economist* 314(7636):43, 1990.

Lutz S: Nurses begin Romanian mission, *Modern Healthcare* 21(34):13, 1990.

Lutz S: US execs find Romanian health system "depraved," *Mod Healthcare* 20(37):2, 1990.

Nolan P, Nolan M: Child of hardship, *Nurs Times* 87(12):16, 1991.

Rudin C et al: HIV-1, hepatitis (A, B, and C) and measles in Romanian children, *Lancet* 336(8730):1592, 1990.

◆ RUSSIA

MAP PAGE (259)

Location: Massive disintegration of the former Soviet Union's Communist party and territory occurred in 1992. Declarations of independence by the republics of Latvia, Estonia, and Lithuania were followed rapidly by other republics. Russia extends from the western Black and Baltic Seas to the Pacific Ocean. Its vast areas of plains and plateaus are relieved by some low mountain ranges.

FORMER SOVIET UNION

Major Languages	Ethnic Groups		Major Religions	
Russian	Russian	52%	Atheist	51%
Ukrainian	Ukrainian	16%	Russian	
Turkish	Uzbeks	5%	Orthodox	31%
Georgian	Other	27%	Muslim	11%
Caucasian			Jewish	3%
			Other	4%

The practice of religion became legal in 1989.

Predominant Sick Care Practices: Biomedical. Holistic, folk, and western medical practices coexist. A complete medical system that focuses on prevention and cure is available only in the larger cities.

Health Care Beliefs: Passive role; acute sick care; health promotion is important. Health promotion practices encourage maternal and child care. Health care addresses acute problems and tertiary care; however, rehabilitation is not emphasized.

Ethnic/Race Specific or Endemic Diseases (In former Soviet Union): ENDEMIC: Chloroquine-sensitive malaria in scattered areas bordering Iran and Afghanistan. RISK: Japanese encephalitis; long-term effects of the 1986 Chernobyl nuclear disaster in the Ukraine, Byelorussia, and the Baltic countries are being monitored.

Health Team Relationships: Health care paraprofessionals (nurses in particular) are under the control of physicians and have no independent roles. Questioning a physician's order is unacceptable. The rigid and highly specialized health care system provides separate hospitals for children and adults. The dividing age is 15. Rural hospitals serve all ages.

Families' Role in Hospital Care: Patients in general hospital units wear street clothes. Family members usually bathe, feed, and comfort the patient, as well as change the bed linen.

Family Dominance Patterns: The male usually assumes the dominant role, and the mother and grandmother share domestic and child health decisions.

Eye Contact Practices: Direct, sustained eye contact is the norm.

Touch Practices: Three kisses on the cheek for greeting and for farewells are common. Touch is an important part of nonverbal communication.

Pain Reactions: People are communicative about pain. Some prefer injections for pain relief.

Birth Rites: Most infants are born in hospitals. A wide range of care may not be available in all areas. Hospitalization lasts approximately 2 weeks, and no visitors are allowed for the first 2 days. The mother and child can be viewed through a glass window to protect them against infection.

Death Rites: The family is told first of a serious prognosis, and they decide if the patient should be informed.

Child Rearing Practices: The child is encouraged to focus on the mother, and may continue to do so throughout life. Children are taught to depend heavily on their parents.

National Childhood Immunizations (Former Soviet Union): BCG at 5 days; DPT-1 at 3 months; DPT-2 at 4 months; DPT-3 at 5 months; DPT booster between 18 and 24 months; DT boosters at 9 and 16 years; OPV-1 at 3 months; OPV-2 at 4 months; OPV-3 at 5 months; OPV boosters at 12 months or between 18 and 24 months, between 7 and 8 years, and at 16 years; measles at 12 months and 6 years; mumps at 15 months.

Other Characteristics: Attempting to control or suppress emotions is considered unfriendly, insincere, and dishonest. Hands clasped above the head is a traditional gesture of friendship. Many establish an area of personal space by displaying an impassive facial expression; however, such demeanor should not be automatically interpreted as unfriendly.

BIBLIOGRAPHY

Bridges LB, Clacy BJ: An American perception of Soviet health care, *Kans Nurse* March:1, 1988.

Condon JC, Yousef F: *An introduction to intercultural communication,* New York, 1975, Macmillan.

Dennis LI: Nursing within the Soviet health care system, *Int Nurs Rev* 32(5):149, 1985.

Galanti GA: *Caring for patients from different cultures,* Philadelphia, 1991, University of Pennsylvania Press.

Kinsey D: The moral and professional role of the Russian nurse, *Nurs Health Care* 13(8):426, 1992.

MacAvoy S: A cross-cultural learning opportunity: USSR, *J Cont Educ Nurs* 19(5):196, 1988.

Prosser MH: *The cultural dialogue,* Washington, DC, 1985, SIETAR.

Samovar LA, Porter RE: *Intercultural Communication: a reader,* Belmont, Calif, 1985, Wadsworth.

Schecter J et al: *Back in the U.S.S.R.,* New York, 1988, Macmillan.

Smith H: *The new Russians,* New York, 1990, Random House.

Storey PB: Emergency medical services in the U.S.S.R., In Schwartz GR, editor: *Principles and practice of emergency medicine,* vol 2, Philadelphia, 1978, Saunders.

Storti C: *The art of crossing cultures,* Yarmouth, Me, 1990, Intercultural Press.

Szwez D: Contributor.

◆ RWANDA

MAP PAGE (261)

Location: This landlocked nation in east Africa has grassy hills and deep valleys that support subsistence farming. It is one of Africa's most densely populated countries with all arable land being used.

Major Languages	Ethnic Groups		Major Religions	
Kinyarwanda	Hutu	90%	Catholic	65%
French	Tutsi	9%	Indigenous	
Kiswahili	Twa		Beliefs	25%
	(Pygmoid)	1%	Protestant	9%
			Muslim	1%

Ethnic/Race Specific or Endemic Diseases: ENDEMIC: Yellow fever; chloroquine-resistant malaria. AIDS case rate is 30.5/100,000 people.

National Childhood Immunizations: BCG at birth; DPT-1 at 3 months; DPT-2 at 4 months; DPT-3 at 5 months; measles at 9 months; OPV-1 at 3 months; OPV-2 at 4 months; OPV-3 at 5 months.

Other Characteristics: Menarche may occur later than 15 years of age. The Tutsi are extremely tall people.

BIBLIOGRAPHY

Adler MW, editor: Statistics from the World Health Organization and the Centers for Disease Control, *AIDS* 6(10):1229, 1992.

Overfield T: *Biologic variation in health and illness,* Menlo Park, Calif, 1985, Addison-Wesley.

◆ ST. KITTS-NEVIS

MAP PAGE (257)

Location: Also known as St. Christopher-Nevis, St. Kitts-Nevis is located in the eastern Caribbean among the northern Leeward Islands. The population is primarily rural and concentrated along the coast.

Major Language	Ethnic Groups		Major Religions	
English	Black	95%	Anglican	65%
	Other	5%	Protestant	20%
			Catholic	15%

Ethnic/Race Specific or Endemic Diseases: AIDS case rate is 17.4/100,000 people.

National Childhood Immunizations: No data located.

BIBLIOGRAPHY

Adler MW, editor: Statistics from the World Health Organization and the Centers for Disease Control, *AIDS* 6(10):1229, 1992.

◆ ST. LUCIA

MAP PAGE (257)

Location: St. Lucia is one of the Windward Islands of the eastern Caribbean. It is a volcanic island, and mountains run from north to south. St. Lucians primarily are descendants of black African slaves. The island has a tropical climate.

Major Languages	Ethnic Groups		Major Religions	
English	Black	90%	Catholic	90%
French Patois	Mixed	6%	Protestant	7%
	East Indian	3%	Anglican	
	White		and Other	3%
	and Other	1%		

Ethnic/Race Specific or Endemic Diseases: RISK: Schistosomiasis. The AIDS case rate is 10.5/100,000 people.

National Childhood Immunizations: No data located.

BIBLIOGRAPHY

Adler MW, editor: Statistics from the World Health Organization and the Centers for Disease Control, *AIDS* 6(10):1229, 1992.

◆ ST. VINCENT AND THE GRENADINES

MAP PAGE (257)

Location: These islands are among the Windward Islands of the eastern Caribbean. St. Vincent has forested mountains and a volcano that became active in 1979, and The Grenadines are a chain of hundreds of little islets. The people are primarily descendants of black African slaves. The climate is hot and humid.

Major Languages	Ethnic Groups		Major Religions	
English	African	95%	Anglican	70%
French Patois	Other	5%	Methodist	15%
			Catholic	10%
			Other	5%

Predominant Sick Care Practices: Biomedical.

Health Team Relationships: Nurses are authoritarian and dominate the patients. Slapping patients is acceptable behavior.

Dominance Patterns: Women are often dominant, especially in the home.

Food Practices and Intolerances: Great quantities of fruits and vegetables are eaten; however, meat rarely is in the diet. Food is cooked outside.

Child Rearing Practices: The pregnancy rate is high because the child mortality rate is high. The percentage of children who die before age 5 is high; 50% die before adulthood. School is voluntary.

National Childhood Immunizations: No data located.

Other Characteristics: No records of births, deaths, or diseases are kept.

BIBLIOGRAPHY

Steel J: Lecture notes, Nursing 309, Nov 13, 1991, University of Connecticut.

◆ SAN MARINO

MAP PAGE (258)

Location: Tiny San Marino is the oldest republic in the world. It has a strong, independent history, even though it is completely surrounded by Italy. Its landlocked location in the Apennine Mountains affords a rugged terrain. People remain citizens and have voting privileges no matter where they live.

Major Language	Ethnic Groups		Major Religions	
Italian	Italo-Sanmarinese	99%	Catholic	99%
	Other	1%	Other	1%

Ethnic/Race Specific or Endemic Diseases: RISK: Lipid metabolism disorders; anxiety; depression; irritable bowel syndrome; stomach-gastritis problems.

BIBLIOGRAPHY

Mamon J, Paccagnella B: Patient counseling by general practitioners: Republic of San Marino's experience, *Health Educ Q* 18(1):135, 1991.

◆ SAO TOME AND PRINCIPE

MAP PAGE (261)

Location: The small volcanic islands are located 150 miles (240 km) off the west coast of Africa in the Gulf of Guinea. São Tomé has dense mountainous jungle, and Principe has jagged mountains.

Major Language	Ethnic Groups		Major Religions	
Portuguese	Portuguese-African	98%	Catholic	80%
			Protestant	10%
	African	2%	Other	10%

Ethnic/Race Specific or Endemic Diseases: ACTIVE: Cholera. **ENDEMIC:** Yellow fever; chloroquine-sensitive malaria.

National Childhood Immunizations: BCG at birth; DPT-1 at 3 months; DPT-2 at 4 months; DPT-3 at 5 months; measles at 9 months; OPV-1 at 3 months; OPV-2 at 4 months; OPV-3 at 5 months.

BIBLIOGRAPHY

No data located.

◆ SAUDI ARABIA

MAP PAGE (262)

Location: Most of the Arabian Peninsula of the Middle East is occupied by Saudi Arabia. The Red Sea and the Gulf of Aqaba lie to the west; the Arabian (Persian) Gulf lies to the east. A mountain range spans the length of the western coastline; east of the mountains is a massive plateau, the Rub Al-Khali (Empty Quarter), that contains the world's largest sand desert.

Major Language	Ethnic Groups		Major Religions	
Arabic	Arab	90%	Muslim	99%
	Afro-Asian	10%	Other	1%

Predominant Sick Care Practices: Biomedical; holistic; magico-religious; traditional. Islamic beliefs and culture pervade all aspects of health care. Although advanced technological medical care is available, many among the nomadic tribes in remote villages favor traditional practices. For example, it is believed that healing by cauterization burns out evil spirits and results in many scars on the body.

Health Care Beliefs: Active involvement; health promotion is important. Nomadic tribes and people in remote areas seek treatment only when they are extremely ill and are possibly beyond curative treatment. Many believe that intrusive procedures, such as injections and intravenous fluids, are more effective. Women hold an inferior social position, and their somatic complaints are often signs of emotional distress.

Ethnic/Race Specific or Endemic Diseases: Dental caries caused by the high consumption of dates and poor oral hygiene is a major problem. ENDEMIC: Chloroquine-sensitive malaria; schistosomiasis. RISK: Trachoma; syphilis; leprosy; filariasis in western Saudi Arabia; cutaneous leishmoniasis in Bisha; cholera in the Jizan district; rickets and malnutrition diseases in rural areas.

Health Team Relationships: Health care professionals and support personnel who are the same sex as the patient are important to male and female patients and may be essential for females. Male nurses may not give direct care or enter the room of an adult female patient who is alone. Some may accept female nurses caring for male patients. Elaborate and prolonged greeting rituals are practiced with polite expressions and inquiries. To avoid conflict or to avoid admitting ignorance, people may say "yes" when they mean "no."

Families' Role in Hospital Care: Most patients have one or more family members or sitters staying with them, and most hospitals provide couches in each room. Family and friends may be demanding of health care personnel to ensure that care and attention are given to the patient. The sitter also expects services from nursing staff.

Dominance Patterns: The husband is the family leader and decision maker. A woman cannot sign an operative consent; two male family members sign for her. The man may answer questions directed to his spouse. He may decide when the family member should eat and bathe, or the female may decide basic care patterns, such as when to bathe, eat, and breastfeed. Extended families live together in the same compound. The Saudi mother is revered, and most sons will seek their mothers' opinion on family issues.

Eye Contact Practices: For a woman, direct eye contact is limited to other women or to family members. Educated Saudis respect direct eye contact as a sign of honesty and integrity. An approximate 2-foot separation permits conversationalists to evaluate each other's pupil responses. Pupils dilate with interest and contract with dislike.

Touch Practices: Males may only touch those women who are in the family. It is common for males to hold hands in public. Handshakes are continued for a lengthy period.

Perception of Time: Time has little meaning except in business. *Enshalla* (as Allah wills), or whenever it happens, is the norm. Social rituals continue, while appointments go by unattended.

Pain Reactions: Pain is expressed verbally and nonverbally and with emotion, especially to the family. Immediate pain relief is desired. A great deal of analgesia may be needed for pain relief. Some patients may wish to remain sufficiently alert to be able to pray. Some Arabic cultures make use of analogies and metaphors to describe their pain.

Birth Rites: The father, grandfather, and many female family members are present for birthing. The father may move into the hospital room after delivery; he will be a constant visitor.

Death Rites: Confronting the patient with a grave diagnosis shatters hope and creates mistrust. It is believed that only God knows the true prognosis, and death is discussed with extreme reluctance. After death the body must be washed by a family member before removal from the hospital or the home. No menstruating female can touch the body because she is unclean and will affect the afterlife of the deceased. Embalming and autopsies are rarely permitted. Females express grief by wailing. Muslim belief forbids organ donations or transplants. Muslim physicians may recommend transfusions to save lives. Cremation is not permitted. For Muslim burial the body is wrapped in special pieces of cloth and buried without a coffin in the ground.

Food Practices and Intolerances: Ramadan fasting is practiced from sunup to sundown. The sick person must receive permission to not fast from the Iman during this month. Lamb and rice are common foods. Fresh fruits and vegetables are included among the more up-to-date people. Pork and alcoholic beverages are forbidden. Food deprivation is considered as a precursor to illness. It is customary to have food or beverages offered several times before accepting.

Infant Feeding Practices: Breastfeeding is the predominant practice, and it continues for an average of 1 year. Nomadic people give infants ghee, a semifluid and clarified form of butter, for the first 3 days of life to lubricate and clean the intestines and to give nourishment. A wet nurse may breastfeed until the mother begins lactating. Older children may be fed powdered goat's or camel's milk.

Child Rearing Practices: If a wife does not produce a son and heir, her husband divorces her. Contraception methods are not used, and women may have 15 or more children. Because of the high infant mortality rate, a welcoming party for an infant is delayed for 3 months. Boys are raised in the female section of the household until they are age 10; then the boys are segregated. Boys and girls are educated separately. A traditional practice that is on the decline is to remove the female clitoris at puberty; the vagina may also be partially sewn up to prevent premarital sex and to curtail the sex drive. Females begin wearing the veil by age 12. Premarital and extramarital sex are strongly forbidden by Islamic law and may be punishable by death.

National Childhood Immunizations: OPV-1 at 3 months; OPV-2 at 4 months; OPV-3 at 5 months; BCG at birth; measles at 9 months; DPT-1 at 3 months; DPT-2 at 4 months; DPT-3 at 5 months; DPT booster at 18 months; DT at 6 years or at entry into school.

Other Characteristics: Religious police *(Matowa)* enforce the legal cultural laws governing segregation of the sexes, dress codes, and the use of alcohol and illegal drugs. Covering the hair is required for women. Polygamy is more common among the older generations and is practiced with the condition that the wives will be treated equally. Hope, optimism, and the positive advantages of treatment should be stressed.

BIBLIOGRAPHY

Adelman MB, Lustig MW: Intercultural communication problems as perceived by Saudi Arabian and American managers. Paper presented to the Intercultural Communication Division of the Western Speech Communication Association, San Jose, Calif, 1981.

al-Nasser AN, Bamgboye EA, Alburno MK: A retrospective study of factors affecting breast feeding practices in a rural community of Saudi Arabia, *East Afr Med J* 68(3):174, 1991.

al-Shammari SA: Help-seeking behavior of adults with health problems in Saudi Arabia, *Fam Pract Res J* 12(1):75, 1992.

Anderson R: Saudi Arabian culture. In On the scene, *Nurs Admin Q* 16(2):20, 1992.

Boyles C, Nordhaugen N: An employee health service in Saudi Arabia, *AAOHN J* 37(11):459, 1989.

Brown BJ: Contributor.

Dahlberg N: Innovative management of acute pain: a collaborative approach. Paper presented at the Second International Middle East Nursing Conference, Irbid, Jordan, April 27, 1992.

Daly E: Personal communication, April 26, 1992.

Davis CF: Culturally responsive nursing management in an international health care setting. In On the scene, *Nurs Adm Q* 16(2):36, 1992.

Galanti GA: *Caring for patients from different cultures,* Philadelphia, 1991, University of Pennsylvania Press.

Green J: Death with dignity: Islam, *Nurs Times* 85(5):56, 1989.

Hall ET: Learning the Arabs' silent language, *Psychol Today* Aug:45, 1979.

Hathout MM: Comment on ethical crises and cultural differences, *West J Med* 139(3):380, 1983.

Meleis AI, Jonsen AR: Medicine in perspective: ethical crises and cultural differences, *West J Med* 138(6):889, 1980.

Racy J: Somatization in Saudi women: a therapeutic challenge, *Br J Psychiatry* 137:212, 1980.

Reizian A, Meleis AI: Arab-Americans' perceptions of and responses to pain, *Crit Care Nurse* 6(6):30, 1986.

Ross HM: Societal/cultural views regarding death and dying, *Top Clin Nurs* 1(1):1, 1981.

Sebai ZA, Bella H: Laying the foundations of good health care, *World Health Forum* 11(4):385, 1990.

Storti C: *The art of crossing cultures,* Yarmouth, Me, 1990, Intercultural Press.

◆ **SENEGAL**

MAP PAGE (260)

Location: Senegal is the westernmost nation in Africa and is located on the Atlantic coast. It consists primarily of a rural population that lives by subsistence farming. The country has one of the best transportation systems in Africa. Much of Senegal is low lying and flat, with differentiated dry and wet seasons.

Major Languages	Ethnic Groups		Major Religions	
French	Wolof	36%	Muslim	92%
Wolof	Fulani	17%	Indigenous	
Pulaar	Serer	17%	Beliefs	6%
Diola	Toucouleur	9%	Christian	2%
Mandingo	Diola			
and Other	and Other	21%		

Ethnic/Race Specific or Endemic Diseases: ENDEMIC: Yellow fever; chloroquine-resistant malaria. RISK: Schistosomiasis.

Death Rites: Muslim belief forbids organ donations or transplants. Muslim physicians may recommend transfusions to save lives. Autopsy is uncommon because the deceased must be buried intact. For Muslim burial the body is wrapped in special pieces of cloth and buried without a coffin in the ground. Cremation is not permitted.

Food Practices and Intolerances: Pork, carrion, and blood are forbidden. Food tends to be spicy. Ramadan fasting is practiced with exemptions for the sick.

National Childhood Immunizations: BCG at birth; DPT-1 at 3 months; DPT-2 at 4 months; DPT-3 at 5 months; measles at 9 months; OPV-1 at 3 months; OPV-2 at 4 months; OPV-3 at 5 months.

Other Characteristics: Children under age 5 who migrate from rural to urban areas continue to have a much higher mortality rate.

BIBLIOGRAPHY

Brockerhoff M: Rural-to-urban migration and child survival in Senegal. *Demography 1990* 27(4):601, 1990.

Fassin D et al: Who consults and where? Sociocultural differentiation in access to health care in urban Africa, *Int J Epidemiol* 17(4):858, 1988.

McEvers NC: Health and the assault on poverty in low income countries, *Soc Sci Med* 14(1):41, 1980.

Ross HM: Societal/cultural views regarding death and dying, *Top Clin Nurs* 1(1):1, 1981.

◆ SEYCHELLES

MAP PAGE (261)

Location: Approximately 100 islands in the Indian Ocean east of Africa and northeast of Madagascar form the Seychelles. Many of the islands are uninhabited coral atolls. The country's culture contains French and African influences.

Major Languages	Ethnic Groups		Major Religions	
English	Black/Mulatto	99%	Catholic	90%
French	Other	1%	Anglican	8%
Creole			Other	2%

National Childhood Immunizations: BCG at birth; DPT-1 at 3 months; DPT-2 at 4 months; DPT-3 at 5 months; DPT booster at 18 months; DT at 6 years; measles at 15 months; OPV-1 at 3 months; OPV-2 at 5 months; OPV-3 at 5 months; OPV booster at 18 months.

BIBLIOGRAPHY

No data located.

◆ SIERRA LEONE

MAP PAGE (260)

Location: This west African coastal nation on the Atlantic has a heavily indented coastline with mangrove swamps, wooded hills, and a plateau inland.

Major Languages	Ethnic Groups		Major Religions	
English	Temne	30%	Indigenous	
Krio	Mende	30%	Beliefs	30%
Mende	Creole		Muslim	30%
Temne	and Other	40%	Christian	10%
			Other	30%

Ethnic/Race Specific or Endemic Diseases: ENDEMIC: Yellow fever; chloroquine-resistant malaria. RISK: Schistosomiasis.

National Childhood Immunizations: BCG at birth; DPT-1 at 3 months; DPT-2 at 4 months; DPT-3 at 5 months; measles at 9 months; OPV-1 at 3 months; OPV-2 at 4 months; OPV-3 at 5 months.

BIBLIOGRAPHY

Williams B, Yumbella F: An evaluation of the training of traditional birth attendants in Sierra Leone and their performance after training, *World Health Organ Offset Publ* (95):35, 1986.

◆ SINGAPORE

MAP PAGE (265)

Location: An island nation off the southeast coast of Malaysia, Singapore is one of the most densely populated areas in the world and is a leading economic power with one of the world's largest ports. Its economic power has contributed to its high standards of health, education, and housing. Most people live in the city of Singapore on the main island.

Major Languages	Ethnic Groups		Major Religions	
Malay	Chinese	77%	Buddhist	70%
Mandarin	Malay	15%	Taoist	14%
Tamil	East Indian	6%	Muslim	9%
English	Other	2%	Hindu	7%

Ethnic/Race Specific or Endemic Diseases: RISK: Japanese encephalitis.

Touch Practices: The head is considered sacred. It is an offense to pat a child on the head. Reaching over the patient's head to pass something to another person may be impolite.

National Childhood Immunizations: DPT at 3 months, 4 months, and 5 months; DPT booster at 18 months; DT at

6 years, 11 years, 15 years, and 17 years; BCG at birth; measles at 12 months; rubella at 11 years. Hepatitis B virus infection is a public health problem. Increases have occurred in immunization rates after a nationwide educational program.

BIBLIOGRAPHY

Boon WH: Child health in Singapore: past, present and future, *J Sing Paediatr Soc* Suppl:4, 1979.

Fong NP, Basir H, Seow A: Awareness and acceptance of hepatitis B vaccination in Clementi, Singapore, *Ann Acad Med Singapore* 19(6):788, 1990.

Kong SG et al: Some aspects of child-rearing practices and their relationship to behavioural deviance, *J Singapore Paediatr Soc* 28(1-2):94, 1986.

Soo KS: My child is ill, what shall I do? *J Singapore Paediatr Soc* 24(1-2):93, 1982.

◆ SOLOMON ISLANDS

MAP PAGE (255)

Location: The islands are located in the Pacific Ocean east of Papua New Guinea. Approximately 90% of the people are Melanesian, and many different local languages are spoken. The population is primarily rural. The land consists of forested mountains and low coral atolls, with 10 large and rugged volcanic islands and four groups of smaller islands.

Major Languages	Ethnic Groups		Major Religions	
English	Melanesian	93%	Christian	95%
Local Languages	Polynesian	4%	Other	5%
	Micronesian	1%		
	European and Other	2%		

Ethnic/Race Specific or Endemic Diseases: ENDEMIC: Chloroquine-resistant malaria.

National Childhood Immunizations: BCG at birth, 7 years, and 14 years; DPT at 3 months, 4½ months, and 6 months; DPT boosters at 7 years and at 14 years; polio at 3 months; 4½ months, and 6 months.

BIBLIOGRAPHY
No data located.

◆ SOMALIA

MAP PAGE (260)

Location: Situated in east Africa along the Gulf of Aden and the Indian Ocean, Somalia is unique for its homogenous language and culture. The majority of people are nomads. The arid, barren land is subject to severe droughts and famine and is currently experiencing a drought that is especially severe. The literacy and life expectancy rates are low.

Major Languages	Ethnic Groups		Major Religions	
Somali	Somali	85%	Sunni	
Arabic	Bantu Groups	5%	Muslim	97%
English	Arab		Other	3%
Italian	and Other	10%		

Predominant Sick Care Practices: Traditional. The use of traditional healers including respected and skilled bone setters is widespread throughout the rural and urban parts of the country. Self-medication, herbal medicines, religious acts, and traditional dances are part of traditional treatment procedures.

Ethnic/Race Specific or Endemic Diseases: ENDEMIC: Yellow fever; chloroquine-resistant malaria. RISK: Schistosomiasis.

Death Rites: Muslim belief forbids organ donations or transplants. Muslim physicians may recommend transfusions to save lives. Autopsy is uncommon because the deceased must be buried intact. Cremation is not permitted. For Muslim burial the body is wrapped in special pieces of cloth and buried without a coffin in the ground.

Food Practices and Intolerances: Pork, carrion, and blood are forbidden. Food tends to be spicy. Ramadan fasting is practiced with exemptions for the sick and for children.

Child Rearing Practices: The practice of female circumcision remains almost universal.

National Childhood Immunizations: OPV at birth; OPV-1 at 40 days; OPV-2 at 70 days; OPV-3 at 100 days; BCG at birth; measles at 9 months; DPT-1 at 40 days; DPT-2 at 70 days; DPT-3 at 100 days.

BIBLIOGRAPHY

Brown Y: Female circumcision, *Can Nurse* Apr:19, 1989.

Ross HM: Societal/cultural views regarding death and dying, *Top Clin Nurs* 1(1):1, 1981.

Yusuf HI et al: Traditional medical practices in some Somali communities, *J Trop Pediatr* 30(2):87, 1984.

◆ SOUTH AFRICA

MAP PAGE (261)

Location: South Africa is situated on the southern tip of Africa. It has the Atlantic on its west and the Indian Ocean on its south and east. The country has four independent states (black republics) created as separatist homelands. Traditionally the races are four separate groups: Whites, Indians (Asians), Coloureds, and Blacks. Since 1990 health services and hospitals have been open to all. Although the black African people are in the majority, the minority white people possess dominance.

Major Languages	Ethnic Groups		Major Religions	
Afrikaans	African	70%	Christian	60%
English	White	18%	Hindu	2%
Zulu	Mixed	9%	Muslim	
Xhosa	East Indian	3%	and Other	38%
Sotho				
and Other				

Predominant Sick Care Practices: Biomedical; magico-religious. Discriminatory health care under apartheid favors white Africans over black Africans. Treatments used by traditional healers may include ashes, amulets, and holy water.

Ethnic/Race Specific or Endemic Diseases: ENDEMIC: Chloroquine-resistant malaria. **RISK:** Schistosomiasis; trachoma.

Health Team Relationships: In race-segregated hospitals, a perceived cultural superiority among nurses is reported.

Infant Feeding Practices: Breastfeeding is widespread.

National Childhood Immunizations: No data located.

Other Characteristics: Violence because of social and political unrest accounts for the highest number of deaths and disabilities among young adults. The United States' finger gestures for *thumbs up* and the *V* held palm are insulting gestures.

BIBLIOGRAPHY

Brokaw T: NBC News, June 17, 1991.

Galanti GA: *Caring for patients from different cultures,* Philadelphia, 1991, University of Pennsylvania Press.

Kuhn L et al: *S Afr Med J* 77(9):471, 1990.

Masipa A: Transcultural nursing in South Africa: prospects for the 1990's, *J Transcult Nurs* 3(1):3, 1991.

Nightingale EO et al: Apartheid medicine: health and human rights in South Africa, *JAMA* 264(16):2097, 1990.

Oldshue R, Shange E, Vost DA: Maternal and child care services in rural Kwazulu, *S Afr Med J* 55(9):344, 1979.

Sutter EE, Ballard RC: A community approach to trachoma control in the Northern Transvaal, *S Afr Med J* 53(16):622, 1978.

Van Der Walt AM: Patient classification in the Groote Schuur Hospital region, Republic of South Africa, *Nurs Admin Q* 16(2):43, 1992.

Westaway MS: Health complaints, remedies and medical assistance in a peri-urban area, *S Afr Med J* 77(1):34, 1990.

◆ SPAIN

MAP PAGE (258)

Location: Spain occupies most of the Iberian Peninsula in southwest Europe. Spain is bordered by the Atlantic on the west and the Mediterranean to the south; Africa is only 10 miles (16 km) away. The Pyrenees Mountains in the northeast separate Spain from France. The Spanish people include groups that are originally from other parts of Europe and from the Mediterranean.

Major Languages	Ethnic Groups		Major Religions	
Castilian Spanish	Spanish	73%	Catholic	99%
Catalan	Catalan	16%	Other	1%
Galician	Galician	8%		
Basque	Basque and Other	3%		

Health Care Beliefs: Health promotion is important. It is believed that disease is caused by an upset in body balance.

Health Team Relationships: School for children is continued in some hospitals. Children do not remain in bed in the hospital unless it is indicated.

Dominance Patterns: The father is the undisputed head of the family. Family ties are strong, and the extended family pattern is prevalent.

Eye Contact Practices: Direct eye contact prevails among the younger generations.

Touch Practices: The tendency is toward touching frequently.

Time Perceptions: People take a casual attitude toward punctuality. An exception is the 1 PM to 4 PM afternoon siesta, which is always observed promptly. Bedtime can be very late.

Food Practices and Intolerances: Spanish food is not spiced liberally; although olive oil is an important ingredient. Breakfast is light, and the main meal is eaten during the afternoon siesta period. An early evening snack is taken, and a several-course dinner is eaten late in the evening.

Child Rearing Practices: Learning the sex role differences begins early. The opportunity to enter a desired field of education is based on passing the competitive qualifying examinations.

National Childhood Immunizations: DPT at 3 months, 5 months, and 7 months; DT at 18 months; tetanus at 6 years and 14 years; OPV at 3 months, 5 months, 7 months, 18 months, 6 years, and 14 years; MMR at 15 months; rubella for girls at 11 years.

Other Characteristics: Women are expected to be loyal to their husbands, yet they are to tolerate extramarital relationships. The influence of the woman extends beyond the home into business, education, and government. The woman's traditional submissive role is currently being modified. The traditional "OK" sign has a vulgar connotation in Spain. Prescriptions are not required for many medications.

BIBLIOGRAPHY

Brigham Young University Language and Intercultural Research Center: *Espana,* Provo, Utah, 1977.

Elsden C, Yarritu C: Development of nursing services in the Basque Autonomous Region, Spain, *Nurs Admin Q* 16(2):68, 1992.

Galanti GA: *Caring for patients from different cultures,* Philadelphia, 1991, University of Pennsylvania Press.

Geissler EM, Dick MJ: Spanish hospitals: personal observations and impressions, *Sigma Theta Tau Reflect* 9:2, 1983.

Giger JN, Davidhizar RE: *Transcultural nursing,* St Louis, 1991, Mosby.

Plata CB: Personal communications, July-August, 1990.

◆ SRI LANKA

MAP PAGE (264)

Location: Sri Lanka formerly Ceylon is an island located just off the southeast tip of India. It has a tropical climate with flat, rolling land and mountains in the southcentral area.

Major Languages	Ethnic Groups		Major Religions	
Sinhala	Sinhalese	74%	Buddhist	69%
Tamil	Tamil	18%	Hindu	15%
English	Moor	7%	Christian	8%
	Other	1%	Muslim	8%

Predominant Sick Care Practices: Biomedical; magico-religious; traditional. Choice of health systems may be based on availability of practitioners. Traditional healers may refer patients to the physician or hospital when it is believed that modern medicine can save the client's life. Mental health problems are believed to be within the realm of indigenous practitioners.

Ethnic/Race Specific or Endemic Diseases: ENDEMIC: Chloroquine-resistant malaria. RISK: Japanese encephalitis.

Dominance Patterns: The male is dominant. Women may be restricted from evening activities. In traditional homes, guests are separated into male and female groups for social interactions.

Health Team Relationships: Patients may consider titles more important than names and use the health professional's title.

Touch Practices: Greeting is done by placing the palms together in a praying motion.

Birth Rites: Most deliveries occur in hospitals.

Death Rites: Preference is for quality over quantity of life because of the Buddhist belief in reincarnation and the expectation of less suffering in the next life. The dying are helped to remember their past good deeds and to achieve a fitting mental state. Autopsies are permitted and cremation is preferred.

Food Practices and Intolerances: The right hand is used for eating, and the left hand is reserved for cleaning oneself after elimination.

Infant Feeding Practices: Early breastfeeding of colostrum is common. Formula is introduced around 6 months.

National Childhood Immunizations: BCG at birth; DPT at 3 months, 5 months, and 7 months; DPT booster at 18 months; measles at 9 months; OPV at 3 months, 5 months, and 7 months; OPV booster at 18 months.

Other Characteristics: Mortality statistics are higher for women than men, apparently because males receive preferential treatment. Elimination is accomplished by squatting over a receptacle on the floor. Toilets with seats may be a safety hazard for people who are unfamiliar with them. It may be preferred that bedpans be placed on the floor because elimination is considered unclean and is not done in bed.

BIBLIOGRAPHY

Caldwell J et al: Sensitization to illness and the risk of death: an explanation for Sri Lanka's approach to good health for all, *Soc Sci Med* 28(4):365, 1989.

Factors that influence patients in Sri Lanka in their choice between Ayurvedic and Western medicine (letter), *Br Med J* 291(6499):899, 1985.

Galanti GA: *Caring for patients from different cultures,* Philadelphia, 1991, University of Pennsylvania Press.

Geissler EM: Personal observations, 1968-1969.

Jeyarajah R: Factors that influence patients in Sri Lanka in their choice between Ayurvedic and Western medicine. Response to article in *Br Med J* 291:899, 1985.

Lally MM: Last rites and funeral customs of minority groups, *Midwife Health Visit Comm Nurse* 14(7):224, 1978.

Nichter M, Nordstrom C: A question of medicine answering health commodification and the social relations of health in Sri Lanka, *Cult Med Psychiatry* 13(4):367, 1989.

Soysa PE, Fernando DN, Abbeywickrama K: Role of health personnel in the promotion of breast feeding practices, *J Trop Pediatr* 34(2):75, 1988.

Thapa S, deSilva V, Farr MG: Potential acceptors of Norplant implants in comparison with recently sterilized women in Sri Lanka, *Fam Health Internal Adv Contraception* 5(3):147, 1989.

Waxler NE: Behavioral convergence and institutional separation: an analysis of plural medicine in Sri Lanka, *Cult Med Psychiatry* 8(2):187, 1984.

Weisfeld GE: Sociobiological patterns of Arab culture, *Ethnolog Sociobiol* 11:23, 1990.

Wolfers I: Factors that influence patients in Sri Lanka in their choice between Ayurvedic and Western medicine. Response to article in *BMJ* 291:970, 1985.

◆ SUDAN

MAP PAGE (260)

Location: This northeast African country (formerly Anglo-Egyptian Sudan) is the largest on the continent. Parts of the Libyan Desert are in the north. The Nile River runs through Sudan, and the southern region and tropical climate support fertile land and forests. African blacks are concentrated in the south, and Arabs are in the central and northern regions. The two cultures are quite distinct. The country is experiencing drought, famine, and civil war.

Major Languages	Ethnic Groups		Major Religions	
Arabic	Black	52%	Sunni Muslim	70%
English	Arab	39%	Indigenous Beliefs	20%
Nubian	Beja	6%	Christian	
Ta Bedawie	Other	3%	and Other	10%
Other				

Predominant Sick Care Practices: Biomedical; magico-religious. Money for biomedical health care is currently being used for the civil war.

Ethnic/Race Specific or Endemic Diseases: ACTIVE: Yellow fever. ENDEMIC: Chloroquine-resistant malaria. RISK: Schistosomiasis.

Death Rites: Muslim belief forbids organ donations or transplants. Muslim physicians may recommend transfusions to save lives. Autopsy is uncommon because the deceased must be buried intact. Cremation is not permitted. For Muslim burial the body is wrapped in special pieces of cloth and buried without a coffin in the ground.

Food Practices and Intolerances: Pork, carrion, and blood are forbidden. Food tends to be spicy. Ramadan fasting is practiced with exemptions for the sick and for children.

Infant Feeding Practices: Many mothers still breastfeed for 1 year; however, a trend toward a shorter duration is occurring among educated women. The belief that children's fluid intake should be reduced and that breastfeeding should be stopped or reduced during episodes of diarrhea is popular.

Child Rearing Practices: Family planning may be perceived as being against the wishes of the husband or against religious teachings.

National Childhood Immunizations: OPV-1 at 3 months; OPV-2 at 4 months; OPV-3 at 5 months.

BIBLIOGRAPHY

Ali BH, Roese PM: Children and youth in a population of the Shendi area, Sudan, *Arztl Jugendkd* 80(3):135, 1989.

Beasley A: Breastfeeding studies: culture, biomedicine, and methodology, *J Hum Lact* 7(1):7, 1991.

El Tom AR et al: Family planning in the Sudan: a pilot project success story, *World Health Forum* 10:333, 1989.

Grotberg EH: Research in Sudan on child and family concerns, *Child Today* 12(5):18, 1983.

Ross HM: Societal/cultural views regarding death and dying, *Top Clin Nurs* 1(1):1, 1981.

Rushwan HE, Ferguson JG, Bernard RP: Hospital counseling in Khartoum: a study of factors affecting contraceptive acceptance after abortion, *Int J Gynaecol Obstet* 15(5):440, 1978.

Zaki V: Personal communication, Sept 28, 1992.

◆ SURINAME

MAP PAGE (258)

Location: Suriname (formerly Dutch Guiana) is situated on the northeast coast of South America. The interior has tropical rain forests, and the narrow coastal area is swampland.

Major Languages	Ethnic Groups		Major Religions	
Dutch	Hindustani	37%	Hindu	27%
English	Creole	31%	Protestant	25%
Sranan Tongo	Javanese	15%	Catholic	23%
Hindustani	Bush Black	10%	Muslim	20%
Javanese	Native American		Other	5%
	and Other	7%		

Ethnic/Race Specific or Endemic Diseases: ENDEMIC: Yellow fever; chloroquine-resistant malaria (in the interior with no risk in urban areas). **RISK:** Schistosomiasis.

National Childhood Immunizations: No data located.

BIBLIOGRAPHY

Rozendaal JA: Epidemiology and control of malaria in Suriname, *Bull Pan Am Health Organ* 25(4):336, 1991.

◆ SWAZILAND

MAP PAGE (261)

Location: Swaziland is landlocked and located near the Indian Ocean side of southern Africa. The climate is temperate.

Major Languages	Ethnic Groups		Major Religions	
English	Swazi	90%	Christian	57%
Siswati	Zulu	2%	Indigenous	
	European	2%	Beliefs	43%
	Other	6%		

Ethnic/Race Specific or Endemic Diseases: RISK: Chloroquine-resistant malaria; schistosomiasis.

Infant Feeding Practices: Mothers often return to work soon after delivery to supplement families' incomes; therefore soft table foods usually are introduced to infants at 6 to 8 weeks. This early introduction may slow the infants' growth.

Child Rearing Practices: Working mothers require alternate care givers. National policy supports an intensive program that monitors and promotes growth in children and works to eliminate stunted growth.

National Childhood Immunizations: BCG at birth; DPT-1 at 3 months; DPT-2 at 4 months; DPT-3 at 5 months; DPT booster at 18 months; measles at 9 months; OPV-1 at 3 months; OPV-2 at 4 months; OPV-3 at 5 months; OPV booster at 18 months. A governmental fee increase has resulted in a decline in protection against childhood diseases.

BIBLIOGRAPHY

Chaudhuri SN: National policy on growth monitoring and promotion: Swaziland leads the way, *Indian J Pediatr Suppl* 55:S106, 1988.

Yoder RA: Are people willing and able to pay for health services? *Soc Sci Med* 29(1):35, 1989.

◆ SWEDEN

MAP PAGE (258)

Location: This northern European country is located in eastern Scandinavia along the Baltic Sea. It is a land of many lakes. Half of Sweden is also covered by forests. Its northern boundary extends into the Arctic Circle. Sweden has one of the world's highest standards of living.

Major Languages	Ethnic Groups		Major Religions	
Swedish	Swedish	93%	Lutheran	94%
Lapp	Lappish	4%	Catholic	1%
Finnish	Finnish	3%	Other	5%

Predominant Sick Care Practices: Biomedical.

Health Care Beliefs: Active involvement; health promotion important. Health promotion is primarily emphasized in maternal and child care. Free universal health care is provided. People are expected to be responsible for self-care and health; however, many social services are available. The focus of care is in health care facilities and not in the community-family setting.

Ethnic/Race Specific or Endemic Diseases: RISK: Sjogren-Larsson syndrome; Krabbe disease; Rett's syndrome; phenylketonuria; alcoholism is widespread and results in severe fetal alcohol syndrome in some infants.

Health Team Relationships: Receptionist nurses who are contacted by telephone are the first point of contact in the health care system. The physician holds an authoritarian role and is not questioned. While patients are expected to say what they feel, the expression of feelings is not encouraged by health care professionals.

Families' Role in Hospital Care: Staff provides for all the patient's needs; however, the family may assist if they like. Flexible visiting hours are observed. Stipends are paid to individuals who provide care for a sick family member at home.

Dominance Patterns: This is an egalitarian society; however, the woman usually is responsible for household chores, food purchases, and food preparation.

Eye Contact Practices: Direct eye contact is observed when speaking.

Touch Practices: This is a society that touches infrequently.

Time Perceptions: Northern Swedes are not as time conscious as those from large cities in southern Sweden. A 15- to 30-minute delay is tolerated. Swedes are present and future oriented and plan for that which may be important in the future.

Pain Reactions: Nonexpressive reactions or expressive reactions to pain are acceptable. To express pain, muscles may be contracted in the body or in the face with accompanying verbal expression. Immediate pain relief is expected.

Birth Rites: Sweden has one of the lowest infant mortality rates. Women may choose any position to deliver, even underwater. ABC Clinics provide many choices for delivery, including father-sibling participation. Under some options the father may cut the umbilical cord, the baby is placed on the mother's abdomen, and the family is left alone for several hours. Rooming in during the day is common. The infant is returned to the nursery at night.

Death Rites: Quiet and open grief are acceptable. The dying person is not to be left alone or without family present. After death a closed coffin is used. The body is not viewed after death.

Food Practices and Intolerances: Breakfast often consists of coffee or tea, a sandwich of meat and cheese, or porridge. A large meal is eaten at lunch and at dinner. Meatballs with potatoes and gravy are popular. Coffee breaks may include a sandwich at midmorning and at midafternoon. Fish, meat, and bananas are foods that are eaten often.

Infant Feeding Practices: Breastfeeding is preferred, is encouraged, and continues for about 1 year. Other foods are introduced at 4 or 5 months. Bottle feeding is discouraged.

Child Rearing Practices: Children are raised in a permissive environment but with safety limits. School starts at age 7. Nurses from government-sponsored day care centers care for the preschool child. Most mothers work.

National Childhood Immunizations: DT at 3 months, 5 months, 12 months, and 10 years; injectable PV at 3 months, 5 months, 12 months, and 6 years; BCG at 5 months to children with high risk; MMR at 18 months and at 12 years.

BIBLIOGRAPHY

Bergh I: Contributor.

Boyle JS, Andrews MM: *Transcultural concepts in nursing care,* Glenview, Ill, 1989, Scott, Foresman/Little, Brown College Division.

Carr C: A four-week observation of maternity care in Finland, *J Obstet Gynecol Neonatal Nurs* 18(2):100, 1989.

Dahlen T: Contributor.

Ekblad S: Influence of child-rearing on aggressive behavior in a transcultural perspective, *Acta Psychiatr Scand Suppl* 344:133, 1988.

Engquist A: Personal communication, August 14, 1992.

Forni PR: Health care delivery in Sweden and Finland: a challenge to the American system, *J Prof Nurs* 2(4):234, 1986.

Geissler EM: Personal observations, August 11-15, 1992.

Granger R: Effects of maternal alcohol/drug use on the infant/child: issues and interventions. Lecture presented at the Hole in the Wall Gang Camp, Ashford, Conn, May 14, 1992.

Marklund B et al: Evaluation of the telephone advisory activity at Swedish primary health care centres, *Fam Pract* 7(3):184, 1990.

Morgensen E: Personal communication, August 13, 1992.

Morris J: Rett's syndrome: a case study, *J Neurosci Nurs* 22(5):285, 1990.

Nettelbladt P, Uddenberg N, Englesson I: Sex-role patterns, paternal rearing attitudes and child development in different social classes, *Acta Psychiatr Scand* 64(1):12, 1981.

Sheehy B: Ideological exchange, *Nurs Times* 86(3):36, 1990.

Solheim JS: A cross-cultural examination of use of corporal punishment on children: a focus on Sweden and the United States, *Child Abuse Negl* 6(2):147, 1982.

Timpka T, Arborelius E: The primary-care nurse's dilemmas: a study of knowledge use and need during telephone conversations, *J Adv Nurs* 15:1457, 1990.

Waldenstrom U, Swenson A: Rooming-in at night in the postpartum ward, *Midwifery* 7(2):82, 1991.

Westbrook MT, Nordholm LA, McGee JE: Cultural differences in reactions to patient behaviour: a comparison of Swedish and Australian health professionals, *Soc Sci Med* 19(9):939, 1984.

Whetstone WR, Hansson AO: Perceptions of self-care in Sweden: a cross-cultural replication, *J Adv Nurs* 14:962, 1989.

◆ SWITZERLAND

MAP PAGE (258)

Location: Switzerland is a landlocked nation of central Europe, and the topography consists of the Alps, glaciers, lakes, and a large plateau where most people reside. Four official languages are used. The rugged landscape does not support much agriculture. Banking and tourism are important industries.

Major Languages	Ethnic Groups		Major Religions	
German	German	65%	Catholic	49%
French	French	18%	Protestant	48%
Italian	Italian	10%	Other	3%
Romansch	Romansch	1%		
	Other	6%		

Predominant Sick Care Practices: Biomedical.

Time Perceptions: The Swiss are punctual.

Food Practices and Intolerances: Plain, hearty food, heavy, filling soups, and cheese dishes are common.

National Childhood Immunizations: BCG and hepatitis B at birth; BCG repeated between 5 and 7 years and 12 and 15 years; DPT at 3 months, 4 months, and 5 months; DT between 15 and 24 months, 5 and 7 years, and 12 and 15 years; OPV at 3 months, 4 months, 5 months, between 15 and 24 months, 5 and 7 years, and 12 and 15 years; MMR between 15 and 24 months and 12 and 15 years.

BIBLIOGRAPHY

Abelin T: Getting health promotion off the ground in Switzerland, *J Public Health Policy* 9(2):284, 1988.

Condon JC, Yousef F: *An introduction to intercultural communication,* New York, 1975, Macmillan.

Language Research Center: *German-speaking people of Europe,* Provo, Utah, 1976, Brigham Young University.

◆ SYRIA

MAP PAGE (262)

Location: One of the world's oldest civilizations, Syria is located at the eastern end of the Mediterranean Sea. The east is desert with coastal plains, fertile lowlands, and mountains in the remainder of the country.

Major Languages	Ethnic Groups		Major Religions	
Arabic	Arab	90%	Sunni Muslim	74%
Kurdish	Kurdish		Other Muslim	16%
Armenian	and Other	10%	Christian	10%
French				
English				

Ethnic/Race Specific or Endemic Diseases: ENDEMIC: Chloroquine-sensitive malaria (no risk in urban areas). RISK: Schistosomiasis.

Families' Role in Hospital Care: Family members or close friends accompany the patient and expect to participate in care or to take a vigilant supervisory role.

Time Perceptions: Planning ahead has the potential of defying God's will. Lack of planning is not an indication of lack of interest.

Pain Reactions: Immediate pain relief is expected and may be persistently requested. The belief in conserving energy for recovery is in conflict with therapies that require exertion. Pain is expressed privately or only with close relatives and friends. The exception occurs during labor and delivery, when pain is expressed vehemently.

Death Rites: Families may insist that loved ones are not to be told about a terminal diagnosis. Muslim belief forbids organ donations or transplants. Muslim physicians may recommend transfusions to save lives. Autopsy is uncommon because the deceased must be buried intact. Cremation is not permitted. For Muslim burial the body is wrapped in special pieces of cloth and buried without a coffin in the ground.

Food Practices and Intolerances: Pork, carrion, and blood are forbidden. Food tends to be spicy. Ramadan fasting is practiced with exemptions for the sick and for children.

National Childhood Immunizations: OPV-1 at 3 months; OPV-2 at 4 months; OPV-3 at 5 months (a conflicting WHO report lists OPV at birth, 2, 3, and 4 months); BCG at birth; measles at 9 months; DPT-1 at 2 months; DPT-2 at 3 months; DPT-3 at 4 months; DPT booster between 18 and 24 months; DT-1 at 6 years or at school entry; DT-2 at 12 years.

Other Characteristics: Hope, optimism, and the positive advantages of treatment should be stressed.

BIBLIOGRAPHY

Green J: Death with dignity: Islam, *Nurs Times* 85(5):56, 1989.

Meleis AI, Sorrell L: Arab American women and their birth experiences, *MCN* 6:171, 1981.

Racy J: Death in an Arab culture: Discussion of the paper, *Ann NY Acad Sci* 871:1969.

Reizian A, Meleis AI: Arab-Americans' perceptions of and responses to pain, *Crit Care Nurse* 6(6):30, 1986.

Ross HM: Societal/cultural views regarding death and dying, *Top Clin Nurs* 1(1):1, 1981.

◆ TANZANIA

MAP PAGE (261)

Location: Tanzania is located in east Africa on the Indian Ocean. Africa's highest point, Mt. Kilimanjaro at 19,340 feet (5895 m), and lowest point, the floor of Lake Tanganyika at −1174 feet (−358 m), are found here. The climate, influenced by altitude, is hot and humid on the coast, arid in the central area, and temperate in the highlands. Tanzania is one of the less-developed countries of the world.

Major Languages	Ethnic Groups		Major Religions	
Swahili	African	99%	Muslim	35%
English	Other	1%	Christian	33%
			Indigenous Beliefs	32%

Predominant Sick Care Practices: Traditional. Traditional healers use evil spirits as part of care.

Health Care Beliefs: Acute sick care; health promotion is important. The trend is toward health promotion among infants and children.

Ethnic/Race Specific or Endemic Diseases: RISK: Cholera; schistosomiasis. **ENDEMIC:** Yellow fever; chloroquine-resistant malaria (including urban areas); tse-tse fly infestation. The AIDS case rate is 29.1/100,000 people.

Dominance Patterns: Because the family, rather than the individual, is valued, language that reflects group ownership, rather than individual ownership, is used. Traditionally the status of women is inferior to that of men. The mother-in-law plays a key role during the wife's pregnancy in some tribes.

Time Perceptions: Time is not a major concern.

Birth Rites: Traditional birth attendants are often used, and many women prefer home births. Abstinence from sexual intercourse during pregnancy is relatively common. A tendency exists to prefer boys over girls. Various tribes may not touch the umbilical cord until it falls off; some may put cow dung on the cord.

Food Practices and Intolerances: Children may drink alcohol freely in a few tribes.

Infant Feeding Practices: Breastfeeding begins with colostrum the first or second day after birth and may continue for 2 to 3 years. Weaning onto a soft maise soup begins at 3 to 4 months.

Child Rearing Practices: A woman's most important role is to bear as many children as possible and to take full responsibility for their care. During the preschool years child care may be shared by female relatives or babysitters. Female circumcision was formerly a common practice in some tribes; therefore surgical scarring of the female genitalia may still be encountered. Traditional females remain indoors for a year during puberty to learn proper behavior; they have limited contact with males. Traditional practices for family planning include breastfeeding, abstinence, and polygamy.

National Childhood Immunizations: BCG at birth; DPT-1 at 1 month; DPT-2 at 2 months; DPT-3 at 3 months; measles at 9 months; OPV-1 at 1 month; OPV-2 at 2 months; OPV-3 at 3 months.

Other Characteristics: An interaction may begin by first establishing a "laughing relationship": one person laughs gently and another echoes the laugh.

BIBLIOGRAPHY

Adler MW, editor: Statistics from the World Health Organization and the Centers for Disease Control, *AIDS* 6(10):1229, 1992.

Condon JC, Yousef F: *An introduction to intercultural communication,* New York, 1975, Macmillan.

Heggenhougen HK: Will primary health care efforts be allowed to succeed? *Soc Sci Med* 19(3):217, 1984.

Mella PP: Effects of educated professionals on the health and care of women in Tanzania, *Health Care Women Int* 8(4):239, 1987.

Pedersen B: A pilot project for training traditional birth attendants, *J Nurse Midwifery* 30(1):43, 1985.

◆ THAILAND

MAP PAGE (265)

Location: Thailand (formerly Siam) is located in the western Indochinese and the northern Malay peninsulas. It enjoys a variety of forested mountains, plateaus, and alluvial valleys with rain forests in its southern peninsula.

Major Languages	Ethnic Groups		Major Religions	
Thai	Thai	75%	Buddhist	95%
English	Chinese	14%	Muslim	4%
	Other	11%	Christian	1%

Predominant Sick Care Practices: Biomedical; magico-religious.

Ethnic/Race Specific or Endemic Diseases: ENDEMIC: Chloroquine- and Fansidar-resistant malaria (no risk in urban areas). RISK: Japanese encephalitis; schistosomiasis; adult lactase deficiency; hemoglobin E disease.

Health Team Relationships: If the Thai suggests a course of action cautiously and hesitantly he or she wants that course of action to be followed. More nurses hold doctoral degrees than other females do in other occupational fields.

Dominance Patterns: Men are dominant, yet women have considerable authority in domestic and commercial aspects of family life. Thai society is structured more on social hierarchy than it is on equality; however, self is perceived as an autonomous individual rather than as part of a family or of an extended group.

Touch Practices: Because the head is considered sacred, it is inappropriate to pat a child on the head. Also, reaching over the patient's head to pass something to another person may be considered impolite.

Birth Rites: The new mother keeps warm regardless of the ambient temperature because of the belief that this will help lactation. In the north it is believed that the wrists must be bound with string to prevent loss of the soul. A common position for birth at home has the husband sitting on the mattress with his knees supporting his wife's shoulders and her head between his thighs. He may stroke her face and hair for emotional support. After delivery the husband buries the placenta. A ritual postpartum month may be observed, and some mothers eat only rice gruel during the first postpartum week.

Death Rites: For those who adhere to Buddhist beliefs of reincarnation, preference is for quality over quantity in life because it is believed that there will be less suffering in the next life. Therefore the dying should be helped to recall their past good deeds and to achieve a fitting mental state. Autopsies are permitted, and cremation is preferred.

Food Practices and Intolerances: Rice is a staple.

Infant Feeding Practices: Breastfeeding is common; however, some indications of decline are apparent. Children are bottlefed supplemental foods and liquids at early ages.

Child Rearing Practices: Grandmothers play an important role in child rearing. Children are taught to be polite, modest, self-controlled, and deferential—values that are espoused in Buddhism.

National Childhood Immunizations: BCG at birth; DPT at 2 months, 4 months, and 6 months; measles at 9 months; OPV at 2 months, 4 months, and 6 months.

Other Characteristics: The higher the hands are held (the norm being chest level), the more respect is shown during greeting; however, if the hands are held above eye level, it is an insult. Because the head is sacred, placing a piece of clothing worn on a lower part of the body on a pillow where the head is to be placed is unacceptable behavior. Pointing your feet at a person is unacceptable. Some prefer injections rather than pills.

BIBLIOGRAPHY

Beardslee C et al: Nursing care of children in developing countries: issues in Thailand, Botswana and Jordan, *Recent Adv Nurs* 16:31, 1987.

Blease DA: The Asian mother and her expectations, *Midwives Chron Nurs Notes* 98(1171):xiii, 1985.

Boyle JS, Andrews MM: *Transcultural concepts in nursing care,* Glenview, Ill, 1989, Scott, Foresman/Little, Brown College Division.

Chayovan N, Knodel J, Wongboonsin K: Infant feeding practices in Thailand: an update from the 1987 demographic and health survey, *Stud Fam Plann* 21(1):40, 1990.

Fungladda W, Sornmani S: Health behavior, treatment-seeking patterns, and cost of treatment for patients visiting malaria clinics in western Thailand, *SE Asian J Trop Med Public Health* 17(3):379, 1986.

Gualtieri V: Preventing is better than fixing, *Amer J Nurs* 91(2):110, 1991.

Horn BM: Cultural concepts and postpartal care, *Nurs Health Care* 2(9):516, 1981. Reprint in *J Transcult Nurs* 2(1):48, 1990.

Lally MM: Last rites and funeral customs of minority groups, *Midwife Health Visit Comm Nurse* 14(7):224, 1978.

Muecke MA: Health care systems as socializing agents: childbearing the north Thai and western ways, *Soc Sci Med* 10:177, 1976.

Muecke MA, Srisuphan W: From women in white to scholarship: the new nurse leaders in Thailand, *J Transcult Nurs* 1(2):21, 1990.

Sikkema M, Niyekawa A: *Design for cross-cultural learning,* Yarmouth, Me, 1987, Intercultural Press.

Stewart EC, Bennett MJ: *American cultural patterns: a cross-cultural perspective,* rev ed, Yarmouth, Me, 1991, Intercultural Press.

Storti C: *The art of crossing cultures,* Yarmouth, Me, 1990, Intercultural Press.

Weisberg DH: Northern Thai health care alternatives: patient control and the structure of medical pluralism, *Soc Sci Med* 16(16):1507, 1982.

Weisz JR et al: Over- and undercontrolled referral problems among children and adolescents from Thailand and the United States: the Wat and Wai of cultural differences, *J Consult Clin Psychol* 55(5):719, 1987.

◆ TOGO

MAP PAGE (260)

Location: Togo (formerly Togoland) is located in west Africa with a small coastline on the Gulf of Guinea. Most of Togo's people are black Africans. Togo consists of mountains and a small coastal plain. The climate is primarily hot and humid.

Major Languages	Ethnic Groups		Major Religions	
French	Ewe	35%	Indigenous Beliefs	70%
Ewe	Kabye	22%	Christian	20%
Mina	Mina	6%	Muslim	10%
Dagomba	Other	37%		
Kabye				
and Other				

Ethnic/Race Specific or Endemic Diseases: ENDEMIC: Yellow fever; chloroquine-resistant malaria (including urban areas). **RISK:** Schistosomiasis. The AIDS case rate is 13/100,000 people.

National Childhood Immunizations: No data located.

BIBLIOGRAPHY

Adler MW, editor: Statistics from the World Health Organization and the Centers for Disease Control. *AIDS* 6(10):1229, 1992.

◆ TONGA

MAP PAGE (255)

Location: Tonga (also called the Friendly Islands) is a series of volcanic and coral islands. Less than one third of the islands are inhabited. The country is located in the western South Pacific northeast of New Zealand. The majority of the population live on the largest island, Tongatapu. It has the highest percentage of arable land of any country in the world. School enrollment is high, and most people are literate. The climate is subtropical.

Major Languages	Ethnic Groups		Major Religions	
Tongan	Polynesian	99%	Catholic	36%
English	Other	1%	Hindu	23%
			Protestant	13%
			Muslim	6%
			Other	22%

Health Care Beliefs: Acute sick care only.

National Childhood Immunizations: DPT at 2 months, 3 months, and 4 months; DT at 5 years; polio at 2 months, 3 months, 4 months, and 5 years; BCG at birth and upon leaving school; measles at 9 months.

Other Characteristics: Raising the eyebrows is a "yes" answer to a question. It is forbidden to do anything outdoors on Sundays.

BIBLIOGRAPHY

Finau SA, Taummoepeau B, To'a L: Review of the village health worker pilot scheme in Tonga, *NZ Med J* 99(807):592, 1986.

Storti C: *The art of crossing cultures,* Yarmouth, Me, 1990, Intercultural Press.

Theroux P: NBC Today Show, June 22, 1992.

◆ TRINIDAD AND TOBAGO

MAP PAGE (257)

Location: Trinidad and Tobago are located in the Caribbean just off the Venezuelan coast. Trinidad is the larger of the two and has the majority of the predominantly black African or East Indian people.

Major Languages	Ethnic Groups		Major Religions	
English	Black	43%	Catholic	36%
Hindi	East Indian	40%	Hindu	23%
French	Mixed	14%	Protestant	13%
Spanish	White	1%	Muslim	6%
	Chinese		Other	22%
	and Other	2%		

Health Care Beliefs: Health promotion is important.

Ethnic/Race Specific or Endemic Diseases: ENDEMIC: Yellow fever. RISK: Dengue fever. The AIDS case rate is 13.5/100,000 people.

Health Team Relationships: Health care administration is often hierarchical, authoritarian, and based on seniority.

Families' Role in Hospital Care: Materials for physical care (food and clean clothing) are expected from male relatives, while emotional support comes from female relatives, especially sisters.

Dominance Patterns: The male is dominant and the female is more yielding.

Time Perceptions: Rewards for current activity are preferred over delayed gratification.

BIBLIOGRAPHY

Adler MW, editor: Statistics from the World Health Organization and the Centers for Disease Control, *AIDS* 6(10):1229 1992.

Boyle JS, Andrews MM: *Transcultural concepts in nurs.ng care,* Glenview, Ill, 1989, Scott, Foresman/Little, Brown College Division.

Green HB: Temporal attitudes in four Negro subcultures, *Studium Generale* 23(6):571, 1970.

Hezekiah J: Colonial heritage and nursing leadership in Trinidad and Tobago, *Image* 20(3):155, 1988.

Hezekiah J: Postcolonial nursing education in Trinidad and Tobago, *Adv Nurs Sci* 12(2):28, 1990.

◆ TUNISIA

MAP PAGE (260)

Location: Tunisia is located in North Africa near the dividing point between the eastern and western Mediterranean Sea. Its people are descendants of several Berber and Arab groups. It is an agricultural country in the wooded fertile north and the central coastal plains. The south becomes more arid toward the Sahara where it reaches -56 feet (-17 m) sea level. Among Arab nations Tunisia is a leader in advocating women's rights.

Major Languages	Ethnic Groups		Major Religions	
Arabic	Arab	98%	Muslim	98%
French	European	2%	Christian	1%
			Jewish	1%

Ethnic/Race Specific or Endemic Diseases: RISK: Schistosomiasis.

Health Team Relationships: A "yes" followed by "N'sha'llah" (Godwilling) reflects a supernatural control over the future and therefore may mean "no."

Families' Role in Hospital Care: Family members or close friends accompany the patient and expect to participate in care or to take a vigilant, supervisory role.

Pain Reactions: Immediate pain relief is expected and may be persistently requested. The belief in conserving energy for recovery is in conflict with therapies that require exertion. Pain is expressed privately or only with close relatives and friends; however, during labor and delivery pain may be expressed vehemently.

Death Rites: Muslim belief forbids organ donations or transplants. Muslim physicians may recommend transfusions to save lives. Autopsy is uncommon because the deceased must be buried intact. Cremation is not permitted. For Muslim burial the body is wrapped in special pieces of cloth and buried without a coffin in the ground.

Food Practices and Intolerances: Ramadan fasting is practiced.

National Childhood Immunizations: OPV-1 at 3 months; OPV-2 at 4 months; OPV-3 at 6 months.

Other Characteristics: Crowding up to be served is a common and accepted behavior. Hope, optimism, and the positive advantages of treatment should be stressed.

BIBLIOGRAPHY

Auerbach LS: Childbirth in Tunisia: implications of a decision-making model, *Soc Sci Med* 16(16):1499, 1982.

Green J: Death with dignity: Islam, *Nurs Times* 85(5):56, 1989.

Reizian A, Meleis AI: Arab-Americans' perceptions of and responses to pain, *Crit Care Nurse* 6(6):30, 1986.

Ross HM: Societal/cultural views regarding death and dying, *Top Clin Nurs* 1(1):1, 1981.

Storti C: *The art of crossing cultures,* Yarmouth, Me, 1990, Intercultural Press.

◆ TURKEY

MAP PAGE (262)

Location: Turkey is a southeast European and southwest Asian (Anatolia) country at the northeast end of the Mediterranean Sea. The Black Sea is to the north and the Aegean Sea is to the west. The European area is hilly, and the central Asian region is a treeless plateau that is rimmed with high mountains. The climate is hot and dry in summer and cold in winter.

Major Languages	Ethnic Groups		Major Religions	
Turkish	Turkish	85%	Muslim	98%
Kurdish	Kurdish	12%	Other	2%
Arabic	Other	3%		

Predominant Sick Care Practices: Biomedical; holistic. The patient may choose a health care system and change if the desired results are not realized.

Health Care Beliefs: Passive role; acute sick care only. People accept treatment passively.

Ethnic/Race Specific or Endemic Diseases: ENDEMIC: Chloroquine-sensitive malaria (including urban areas); leishmaniasis; trachoma (along the Mediterranean and in the southeast); regional typhoid fever; viral hepatitis. RISK: Goiter; dental problems.

Health Team Relationships: Most physicians are male and have absolute authority. Patients do not question physicians. They do not want to bother him or take his time. Patients usually comply with physician orders if the physician's good will is apparent. Professional dialogue rarely occurs between doctors and nurses. Most nurses are female. Women prefer a nurse or midwife for discussions about family planning.

Families' Role in Hospital Care: A family member usually stays with the patient day and night and provides all care except food preparation.

Dominance Patterns: Decisions generally are made by males. Women are perceived as having lower status in society. Women (especially older women) are the quietly dominant decision makers in their homes, especially when health care decisions are necessary. Husbands are responsible for the paperwork, such as filling out insurance forms.

Eye Contact Practices: Sustained eye contact with authority figures is considered impolite and disrespectful by traditional groups.

Touch Practices: No physical contact occurs during greetings among health care professionals and patients. The abdomen and part of the legs are covered for gynecologic examinations. Outside the health care environment, kissing the cheek and handshaking is customary for greetings.

Time Perceptions: A relaxed attitude is taken toward time.

Pain Reactions: Tolerating and keeping quiet about pain is a common trend. It is regarded as a part of life.

Birth Rites: In rural areas approximately half of the babies are born in some type of health institution; however, in urban areas approximately three fourths of the babies are born in health institutions. The majority of deliveries are assisted by health personnel, official or traditional midwives, or experienced women in rural areas and by physicians or midwives in urban areas. A kneeling position and a prone position on a flat surface are the most common delivery positions. Relatives are not allowed in the hospital's delivery room. Relatives and neighbors help with housework and baby care for 40 days post partum.

Death Rites: Muslim belief forbids organ donations or transplants. Muslim physicians may recommend transfusions to save lives. Autopsy is uncommon because the deceased must be buried intact. Burial is in the ground and is done the day of death or the next day. Time of burial depends on the amount of paperwork involved or on the arrival time of close relatives. Cremation is not permitted. For Muslim burial the body is wrapped in special pieces of cloth and buried without a coffin in the ground.

Food Practices and Intolerances: People along the Black Sea consume a great deal of cabbage. Pork is a forbidden food, and fish and seafood usually are not eaten. Legumes, vegetables, and bread are food staples. Three meals per day is routine. Breakfast is the main meal in rural areas, and dinner is the main meal in urban areas. Ramadan fasting is practiced with exemptions for the sick and for children.

Infant Feeding Practices: Approximately 95% of babies are breastfed until they are 10 to 12 months old. Boys are breastfed longer because of a belief that breastfeeding will make them stronger. Working mothers may only breastfeed for 4 to 6 months. Plain, fresh yogurt, fresh fruit juices, fruit puree, vegetable soup, and soups with grains are advocated for babies who are age 4 to 5 months. Mothers may choose to begin with other solid foods, such as stew broth, rice, or plain cookies.

Child Rearing Practices: The mother is the primary child care giver; however, the paternal grandmother is an important influence. Strict discipline is practiced. Permissive attitudes exist toward boys, and girls are taught to become productive, hard workers. Females start helping with household chores when they enter school.

National Childhood Immunizations: BCG at birth and repeated every 5 years with PPD test; measles at end of 8 (rural) to 12 (urban) months; measles booster at 15 months; OPV-1 at 2 months; OPV-2 at 4 months; OPV-3 at 6 months; OPV booster at 18 to 24 months; DPT-1 at 2 months; DPT-2 at 4 months; DPT-3 at 6 months; DPT booster at 18 to 24 months; DT at 6 years or at entry into school; tetanus toxoid at 10 years.

Other Characteristics: Children commonly believe in the evil eye. Mothers may pin an evil eye pin on the child's shoulder or may say short prayers for protection.

BIBLIOGRAPHY

Akaslan S, Akasian I: Cutaneous leishmaniasis in Sanli Urfa, *Turkiye Parazitoioji Dergisi, Acta Parasitol Turcica* 13(304):43, 1989.

Erefe I: Turkey faces the challenge of Alma-Ata, *Int Nurs Rev* 31(6):169, 1984.

Institute of Population Studies: *Turkish population and health survey,* Ankara, Turkey, 1989, Hacettepe University.

Platin N: Contributor.

Ross HM: Societal/cultural views regarding death and dying, *Top Clin Nurs* 1(1):1, 1981.

Saglik Hizmetleri, Saglik Bakanligi Arastirma Planlama ve Koordinasyon Kurulu Baskanligi, 535:23, 1989.

Sahin ST: Setting up a maternal child health center: organizational and marketing strategies, *Issues Comp Pediatr Nurs* 9:315, 1986.

Turkiye'de Anne ve Cocuklarin Durum Analizi. Ulke Programi 1991-1995, seri no. 2, Yenicag Matbaasi, 1991.

Uyer G: Effect of nursing approach in understanding of physicians' directions, by the mothers of sick children in an out-patient clinic, *Int J Nurs Stud* 23(1):79, 1986.

Uyer G: Health for all and nursing in Turkey, *Int Nurs Rev* 34(1):15, 1987.

◆ TUVALU

MAP PAGE (255)

Location: Located just south of the equator in the western Pacific, Tuvalu (formerly the Ellice Islands) is a chain of nine small islands. The people are Polynesian and live in rural villages. Most of the islands are low atolls about 6 feet (1.8 m) above sea level with surrounding lagoons. The country has a tropical climate.

Major Languages	Ethnic Groups		Major Religions	
Tuvaluan	Polynesian	96%	Christian	90%
English	Other	4%	Other	10%

National Childhood Immunizations: BCG at birth and 6 years; measles at 9 months; DPT at 3 months, 5 months, and 9 months; DPT booster at 6 years; polio at 3 months, 5 months, 9 months, and 6 years.

BIBLIOGRAPHY

Discovery Channel: Natural world, March 30, 1992.

◆ UGANDA

MAP PAGE (261)

Location: Situated in central Africa straddling the equator, this landlocked country consists of swampy lowlands, a fertile plateau, a high mountain range, and desert. It is primarily an agricultural nation, with a temperature that is influenced by changes in altitude.

Major Languages	Ethnic Groups		Major Religions	
English	African	99%	Catholic	33%
Luganda	Other	1%	Protestant	33%
Swahili			Indigenous	
Bantu Languages			Beliefs	18%
Nilotic Languages			Muslim	16%

Ethnic/Race Specific or Endemic Diseases: RISK: Guinea-worm; anemia affects an estimated 70% of Ugandan women; schistosomiasis. **ENDEMIC:** Yellow fever; chloroquine-resistant malaria (including urban areas). The AIDS case rate is 44.9/100,000 people.

Families' Role in Hospital Care: Bathing, bed changing, and meals are provided by the family. Mothers may sleep under the beds of sick children.

Dominance Patterns: The status of the woman depends on her childbearing potential. Polygamy is acceptable, especially if the woman is infertile or if she has passed her childbearing years.

Child Rearing Practices: The husband would reject a wife who practiced birth control.

National Childhood Immunizations: BCG at birth; DPT-1 at 3 months; DPT-2 at 4 months; DPT-3 at 5 months; measles at 9 months; OPV-1 at 3 months; OPV-2 at 4 months; OPV-3 at 5 months.

BIBLIOGRAPHY

Adler MW, editor: Statistics from the World Health Organization and the Centers for Disease Control, *AIDS* 6(10):1229, 1992.

Anderson SR et al: AIDS education in rural Uganda: a way forward, *Int J STD AIDS* 1(5):335, 1990.

Blair J: Health teaching in the context of culture: nursing in East Africa, *Kans Nurse* 6(4):4, 1991.

Lambert H: Care of sick children in Uganda: a personal experience, *Midwife Health Visitor Comm Nurse* 24(7):293, 1988.

Utley G: Report of the Amsterdam Conference on AIDS, NBC News, July 18, 1992.

◆ UNITED ARAB EMIRATES

MAP PAGE (262)

Location: Situated on the eastern side of the Arabian Peninsula, the country is primarily desert and rich in oil. It has one of the highest-per-capita incomes in the world.

Major Languages	Ethnic Groups		Major Religions	
Arabic	Emirian	19%	Muslim	96%
English	Other Arab	23%	Other	4%
Farsi	Asian	50%		
Hindi	Other	8%		
Urdu				

Ethnic/Race Specific or Endemic Diseases: ENDEMIC: Chloroquine-sensitive malaria.

Families' Role in Hospital Care: Family members or close friends accompany the patient and expect to participate in care or to take on a vigilant, supervisory role.

Pain Reactions: Immediate pain relief is expected and may be persistently requested. The belief in conserving energy for recovery is in conflict with therapies that require exertion. Pain is expressed privately or only with close relatives and friends; however, during labor and delivery pain is expressed vehemently.

Death Rites: Muslim belief forbids organ donations or transplants. Muslim physicians may recommend transfusions to save lives. Autopsy is uncommon because the deceased must be buried intact. Cremation is not permitted. For Muslim burial the body is wrapped in special pieces of cloth and buried without a coffin in the ground.

Food Practices and Intolerances: Pork, carrion, and blood are forbidden. Food tends to be spicy. Ramadan fasting is practiced with exemptions for the sick and for children.

National Childhood Immunizations: OPV-1 at 2 months; OPV-2 at 4 months; OPV-3 at 6 months; OPV booster between 6 and 8 years.

Other Characteristics: Hope, optimism, and the positive advantages of treatment should be stressed.

BIBLIOGRAPHY

Green J: Death with dignity: Islam, *Nurs Times* 85(5):56, 1989.

Reizian A, Meleis AI: Arab-Americans' perceptions of and responses to pain, *Crit Care Nurse* 6(6):30, 1986.

Ross HM: Societal/cultural views regarding death and dying, *Top Clin Nurs* 1(1):1, 1981.

◆ UNITED KINGDOM

MAP PAGE (258)

Location: The United Kingdom is European and is primarily located between the Atlantic Ocean and the North Sea. It consists of England, Scotland, Wales, and Northern Ireland. The climate is temperate.

Major Languages	Ethnic Groups		Major Religions	
English	English	82%	Anglican	85%
Welsh	Scottish	10%	Catholic	8%
Gaelic	Irish	2%	Presbyterian	5%
	Welsh	2%	Other	2%
	Asian and Other	4%		

Predominant Sick Care Practices: Biomedical. Alternative medical care (acupuncture, chiropractic, homeopathic, naturopathic, and osteopathic care) may be sought for some health care problems.

Health Care Beliefs: Acute sick care; health promotion is important. Although health promotion is strongly advocated, physicians in some areas may not actively incorporate these beliefs.

Ethnic/Race Specific or Endemic Diseases: RISK: The death rate from coronary heart disease is one of the highest in the world.

Health Team Relationships: Clients may consider titles more important than names and may use the health professional's title when addressing them.

Dominance Patterns: In England the father is traditionally the head of the family, and his authority may not be questioned.

Eye Contact Practices: Staring is believed to be a part of good listening. Understanding is indicated by blinking the eyes.

Touch Practices: The English have generally low touch practices.

Perceptions of Time: The past is valued, and traditional approaches to healing are preferred over new procedures or medications.

Time Perceptions: The English have a strong sense of tradition and aristocracy.

Food Practices and Intolerances: Organ meats are common in England.

Child Rearing Practices: In English families where the father is the authority, the children are obedient.

National Childhood Immunizations: DPT at 2 months, 3 months, 4 months; DP between 4 and 5 years; tetanus between 14 and 17 years; OPV at 2 months, 3 months, 4 months, 4 to 5 years, and 14 to 17 years; MMR between 12 and 15 months; rubella for girls between 10 and 14 years; BCG at 13 years. Northern Ireland has lower immunization rates.

Other Characteristics: The English do not use space as a refuge from others; they set up internalized barriers to withdraw.

BIBLIOGRAPHY

Bingham S: Dietary aspects of a health strategy for England, *BMJ* 303:353, 1991.

Coulter A, Schofield T: Prevention in general practice: the views of doctors in the Oxford region, *Br J Gen Pract* 41(345):140, 1991.

Galanti GA: *Caring for patients from different cultures,* Philadelphia, 1991, University of Pennsylvania Press.

Giger JN, Davidhizar RE: *Transcultural nursing,* St Louis, 1991, Mosby.

Gott M, O'Brien M: Health promotion: practice and the prospect for change, *Nurs Stand* 5(3):30, 1990.

Gott M, O'Brien M: Policy for health promotion, *Nurs Stand* 5(1):30, 1990.

Grove CL: *Communications across cultures,* Washington, DC, 1976, National Education Association.

Hall ET, Hall MR: *Understanding cultural differences,* Yarmouth, Me, 1989, Intercultural Press.

Martinelli AM: Pain and ethnicity: how people of different cultures experience pain, *AORN J* 46(2):273, 1987.

Mead M: *A case history in cross-national communications.* In *The communication of ideas,* New York, 1948, Harper & Row.

O'Gorman F: Business as usual, *Nurs Times* 86(44):62, 1990.

Price P: Health promotion: health visiting in the field, *Nurs Stand* 5(31):53, 1991.

Prosser MH: *The cultural dialogue,* Washington, DC, 1985, SIETAR.

Samovar LA, Porter RE: *Intercultural communication: a reader,* Belmont, Calif, 1985, Wadsworth.

Smith WC et al: Development of coronary prevention strategies by health authorities in the United Kingdom, *Community Med* 11(2):108, 1989.

Thomas KJ et al: Use of nonorthodox and conventional health care in Great Britain, *BMJ* 302(6770):207, 1991.

Wardle J, Steptoe A: The European Health and Behaviour Survey: rationale, methods and initial results from the United Kingdom, *Soc Sci Med* 33(8):925, 1991.

◆ URUGUAY

MAP PAGE (258)

Location: Located on the Atlantic Ocean in southern South America, Uruguay has low, rolling, and fertile grassy plains in the south with plateaus in the north. The climate is temperate, and the winter and summer seasons are opposite those in the northern hemisphere.

Major Languages	Ethnic Groups		Major Religions	
Spanish	White	88%	Catholic	66%
	Mestizo	8%	Protestant	2%
	Black	4%	Jewish	2%
			Unaffiliated and Other	30%

National Childhood Immunizations: DPT-1 at 3 months; DPT-2 at 4 months; DPT-3 at 5 months; OPV-1 at 3 months; OPV-2 at 4 months; OPV-3 at 5 months; OPV boosters at 1 year and 5 years; measles at 1 year; BCG at birth, 5 years, and 12 years.

BIBLIOGRAPHY

No data located.

◆ VANUATU

MAP PAGE (255)

Location: Vanuatu (formerly the New Hebrides) is a collection of about 80 islands in the southwest Pacific Ocean. Much of the land is covered with dense forests.

Major Languages	Ethnic Groups		Major Religions	
Bislama	Melanesian	94%	Christian	90%
French	French	4%	Other	10%
English	Other	2%		

Child Rearing Practices: Education is not compulsory; however, most children attend primary school.

National Childhood Immunizations: DPT at 6 weeks, 10 weeks, and 14 weeks; DT at 6 and 12 years; polio presumably on same schedule as DPT; polio boosters at 6 and 12 years; BCG at birth, 6 years, and 12 years; measles at 9 months.

BIBLIOGRAPHY
No data located.

◆ VENEZUELA

MAP PAGE (258)

Location: Venezuela is located on the Caribbean coast of South America. The climate is tropical, but it is influenced by changes in altitude from the coastline, over the plains and high plateaus, to the Andes Mountains.

Major Languages	Ethnic Groups		Major Religions	
Spanish	Mestizo	67%	Catholic	96%
Indian Languages	White	21%	Protestant	2%
	Black	10%	Other	2%
	Native American	2%		

Ethnic/Race Specific or Endemic Diseases: ENDEMIC: Yellow fever; chloroquine-resistant malaria (with no risk in urban areas). RISK: Dengue fever.

National Childhood Immunizations: DPT-1 at 2 months; DPT-2 at 4 months; DPT-3 at 5 months; DPT booster at 1 year; OPV-1 at 2 months; OPV-2 at 4 months; OPV-3 at 6 months; OPV booster at 1 year; measles at 9 months; BCG at birth.

BIBLIOGRAPHY

No data located.

◆ VIETNAM

MAP PAGE (265)

Location: Located on the Indochinese peninsula in southeast Asia, Vietnam is long and narrow. Most of the country is covered with mountains and plateaus with the marshy Mekong River delta located in the south.

Major Languages	Ethnic Groups		Major Religions	
Vietnamese	Vietnamese	87%	Buddhist	60%
French	Chinese	3%	Confucianist	13%
Chinese	Other	10%	Taoist	12%
English			Catholic	3%
Khmer			Other	12%

Predominant Sick Care Practices: Magico-religious; eastern medicine. Herbal medicine is an important practice; most are classified as *cool,* while most western medicines are considered *hot.* Traditionally illness is dealt with through self-care and self-medication. Folk remedies include variations of acupuncture, massage, herbal remedies, and dermabrasive practices, such as cupping, pinching, rubbing, and burning.

Health Care Beliefs: Acute sick care only. Practices such as pinching or scratching the area let the *bad winds* or the unhealthy air currents out of the body and restore health-producing marks or red lines. Being given medicine that will restore the yin-yang balance and the hot-cold equilibrium is important.

Ethnic/Race Specific or Endemic Diseases: RISK: Cholera; plague; chloroquine-resistant malaria.

Health Team Relationships: Health professionals are considered authority figures and experts, and patients are told little about their conditions, about medicines, or about diagnostic procedures. Therefore, patients may be poor historians. Sparing someone's feelings is more important than truth, so a "yes" may actually mean "no." In traditional families the oldest male makes decisions about health care.

Families' Role in Hospital Care: The patient is considered a person who needs to be taken care of by all family members.

Dominance Patterns: The extended family is the basic unit and consists of three or four generations living together. Decision making is influenced by the astrologic/lunar calendar. Although women defer to men, frequently they control the men, the home, the family's health care, and the economic power of their community. An intense identification of self as part of the family and village minimizes the incentive to excel as an individual. Until they die elderly parents are cared for by children.

Eye Contact Practices: Blinking means only that a message has been received. Looking directly into another's eyes when talking is considered disrespectful.

Touch Practices: The head is considered the seat of the soul and should not be touched. Only the elderly are allowed to touch the heads of young children. Touching persons of the same sex is acceptable. The female breast is accepted dispassionately as the means of infant feeding; however, the lower torso is extremely private. The area between waist and knees is kept covered, even in private. Handshaking has gained wide acceptance with men but not with women. A man will not extend his hand in handshake to a woman or a superior. Sisters and brothers do not touch or kiss each other.

Time Perceptions: Time is viewed as a recurring circle rather than as moving in a linear direction.

Pain Reactions: Pain may be severe before relief is requested.

Birth Rites: Beliefs may include avoiding weddings and funerals and abstaining from sexual intercourse during pregnancy because harm may come to the mother and baby. The squatting position is preferred for delivery. Some type of blooming (such as closed flowers opening) may be used symbolically to help open the cervix during labor. The presence of a female friend may be desired during delivery. Regardless of the temperature the laboring woman drinks only warm or hot water and keeps warm by wearing socks and using blankets. In rural areas, delivery at home with a midwife is preferred. Men, unmarried women, young girls, and the husband are not present during birth. Hot coals may be placed under the bed after delivery. At birth the child is thought to be 1 year old. Circumcision is generally unknown. The newborn should not be given compliments, such as being called beautiful, healthy, or smart, for fear of capture by evil spirits.

Death Rites: Preference is for quality of life over length of life because of beliefs in reincarnation and the expectation that there will be less suffering in the next life. Therefore the dying should be helped to recall their past good deeds and to achieve a fitting mental state. Autopsies are permitted and cremation is preferred. Death at home is preferred over death in the hospital. Upon death the body is washed and wrapped in clean white sheets. The wife may prefer to do this to ensure that the rituals are properly conducted. In some areas a coin or jewels (a wealthier family) and rice (a poorer family) will be put in the mouth of the deceased in the belief that these will help the soul go through the encounters with gods and devils and the soul will be born rich in the next life. Relatives sew small pillows that are placed under the neck, feet, and wrists of the deceased. The body is placed in a coffin, and burial is in the ground.

Infant Feeding Practices: Because colostrum may be perceived as bad milk, bottle feeding may be used until the breasts fill. Breastfeeding may continue for 2 years.

Child Rearing Practices: Methods for calculating the age of an infant may vary as much as 2 years. Parents are relaxed about and enjoy the development of young children. At approximately age 6 strict upbringing begins, independence is discouraged, and parents demand obedience. The oldest child, boy or girl, is responsible for younger siblings if the parents are dead, old, or ill.

National Childhood Immunizations: BCG at birth, 6 years, and 15 years; measles at 9 months; DPT between 3 and 4 months, 5 and 6 months, and 7 and 8 months; DPT booster at 2 years; DT at 6 years; tetanus at 15 years; polio between birth and 12 months and at 2 years, 3 years, 4 years, and 5 years.

Other Characteristics: Belief that illness needs to be drawn out of the body is practiced through coin rubbing. A heated coin or one smeared with oil is vigorously rubbed over the body, producing red welts. The red marks are evidence of the illness being brought to the surface of the body; it is believed that the red marks will occur only in people who are ill to begin with. Because of stigma against mental illness, emotional disturbances may be manifested somatically. Offensive behaviors include a male stranger touching a female, feet on furniture, and photographs of three people in a group. Names are listed in order by family name, middle name, and given name. Legally women retain their own names after marrying. Age is associated with wisdom and experience. It is valued and respected. The American signal to beckon another with the finger or the palm of the hand up is offensive because this is the motion used to call a dog.

BIBLIOGRAPHY

Anderson LK: Intercultural communication between Vietnamese and Americans, Unpublished paper, 1988.

Bates B, Turner AN: Imagery and symbolism in the birth practices of traditional cultures, *Birth* 12(1):29, 1985.

Boyle JS, Andrews MM: *Transcultural concepts in nursing care,* Glenview Ill, 1989, Scott, Foresman/Little, Brown College Division.

Clark MJ: *Nursing in the community,* Norwalk Conn, 1992, Appleton & Lange.

D'Avanzo CE: Barriers to health care for Vietnamese refugees, *J Prof Nurs* 8(4):245, 1992.

Eisenbruch M: Cross-cultural aspects of bereavement. II. Ethnic and cultural variations in the development of bereavement practices, *Cult Med Psychiatry* 8(4):315, 1984.

Galanti GA: *Caring for patients from different cultures,* Philadelphia, 1991, University of Pennsylvania Press.

Horn BM: Cultural concepts and postpartal care, *Nurs Health Care* 2(9):516, 1981.

Lally MM: Last rites and funeral customs of minority groups, *Midwife Health Visit Comm Nurse* 14(7):224, 1978.

Lawson LV: Culturally sensitive support for grieving parents, *MCN* 15:76, 1990.

Li GR: *Funeral practices,* New York, World Relief, n.d.

Marchione J, Stearne SJ: Ethnic power perspectives for nursing, *Nurs Health Care* 11(6):296, 1990.

Muecke MA: Caring for Southeast Asian refugee patients in the USA, *Am J Public Health* 73(4):431, 1983.

Nguyen A, Bounthinh T, Mum S: *Folk medicine, folk nutrition, superstitions,* Washington, DC, 1980, Team Associates.

Rieu LT: *Modern and traditional medical practices of Vietnam: Vietnamese concepts of illness and treatment,* San Francisco, Calif, Indochinese Mental Health Project, n.d.

Rosenberg J, Givens S: Teaching child health care concepts to Khmer mothers, *J Comm Health* 3:157, 1986.

Schreiner D: S.E. Asian folk healing practices/child abuse? Indochinese Health Care Conference, Eugene, Ore, 1981.

Stewart EC, Bennett MJ: *American cultural patterns: a cross-cultural perspective,* rev ed, Yarmouth, Me, 1991, Intercultural Press.

Uland E, Smith S: Southeast Asian mental health issues, Unpublished paper, 1984.

US Department of Health, Education, and Welfare Social Security Administration Office of Family Assistance SSA 77-21013, *A guide to two cultures: Indochinese,* Washington, DC, n.d.

Vandeusen J et al: South East Asian social and cultural customs: similarities and differences, *J Refugee Resettlement* 1:20, 1980.

◆ WESTERN SAMOA

MAP PAGE (255)

Location: Western Samoa, not to be confused with nearby American Samoa, is the larger and western part of the Samoan archipelago and is located approximately halfway between Hawaii and New Zealand.

Major Languages	Ethnic Groups		Major Religions	
Samoan	Samoan	88%	Protestant	70%
English	Euronesian	7%	Catholic	20%
	Other	5%	Other	10%

Predominant Sick Care Practices: Traditional. Technologically advanced equipment and supplies are not readily available, even in urban areas. Coconut oil is a common treatment for many minor problems.

Ethnic/Race Specific or Endemic Diseases: RISK: Injuries from fishing and plantation work accidents; malnutrition from lack of vegetables; hypertension; obesity; diabetes.

Health Team Relationships: Nurses may be referred to as "doctor" in villages without a physician. Hospitals are used primarily for emergencies.

Families' Role in Hospital Care: Family members help care for hospitalized patients, and the facility may provide living quarters for the family.

Dominance Patterns: Male dominance is common; however, it is not universal. The extended family is a strong social force.

Food Practices and Intolerances: Prayers and hymns are said before the evening meal. Taro, green bananas, and breadfruit are dietary staples. Coconut cream is used often for preparing foods. A larger, heavier body build is valued.

National Childhood Immunizations: Samoa: DPT at 3 months, 6 months, and 9 months; DT at 6 years; polio at 3 months, 6 months, and 9 months; BCG at birth; measles at 9 months.

Other Characteristics: Tattoos symbolize manhood but are worn by both sexes. Homes built on raised platforms and open on all sides are designed for tropical weather. Sitting cross-legged for extended periods of time is common. Religion is an important part of all aspects of life, and Sundays are kept as days of rest and relaxation.

BIBLIOGRAPHY

Moyle RM: Sexuality in Samoan art forms, *Arch Sex Behav* 4(3):227, 1975.

Shimamoto Y, Ishida D: The elderly Samoan, *Public Health Nurs* 5(4):219, 1988.

Villafuerte A: Samoa: Reflections on a cultural adventure, *Courier* (Teachers College, Columbia University Nursing Editors Alumni Association Publication) 60:1,3, 1992.

◆ YEMEN

MAP PAGE (262)

Location: Yemen (formerly Yemen and the Yemen Arab Republic) is located on the southwest end of the Arabian Peninsula along the Red Sea and Arabian Sea. In the drier east the land is arid and supports subsistence farming and nomadic herding. In the more heavily populated west, agriculture is the main economy with fertile highlands. The highest point is 12,000 feet (3660 m).

Major Languages	Ethnic Groups		Major Religions	
Arabic	Arab	95%	Muslim	98%
	East Indian		Other	2%
	and Other	5%		

Ethnic/Race Specific or Endemic Diseases: ENDEMIC: Chloroquine-sensitive malaria. RISK: Tuberculosis; schistosomiasis.

Families' Role in Hospital Care: Family members or close friends accompany the patient and expect to participate in care or to take on a vigilant, supervisory role.

Pain Reactions: Immediate pain relief is expected and may be persistently requested. The belief in conserving energy for recovery is in conflict with therapies that require exertion. Pain is expressed privately or with close relatives and friends. During labor and delivery pain is expressed vehemently.

Birth Rites: Infant mortality rate is high.

Death Rites: Muslim belief forbids organ donations or transplants. Muslim physicians may recommend transfusions to save lives. Autopsy is uncommon because the deceased must be buried intact. Cremation is not permitted. For Muslim burial the body is wrapped in special pieces of cloth and buried without a coffin in the ground.

Food Practices and Intolerances: Pork, carrion, and blood are forbidden. Food tends to be spicy. Ramadan fasting is practiced with exemptions for the sick and for children.

National Childhood Immunizations: OPV-1 at 2 months; OPV-2 at 3 months; OPV-3 at 5 months for the part of the country formerly just Yemen. OPV-1 at 6 weeks; OPV-2 at 2 months; OPV-3 at 3 months in the part of the country formerly known as Yemen Arab Republic.

Other Characteristics: Hope, optimism, and positive advantages of treatment should be stressed.

BIBLIOGRAPHY

Green J: Death with dignity: Islam, *Nurs Times* 85(5):56, 1989.
Lambeth S: Health care in the Yemen Arab Republic, *Int J Nurs Stud* 25(3):1, 1988.
Reizian A, Meleis AI: Arab-Americans' perceptions of and responses to pain, *Crit Care Nurse* 6(6):30, 1986.
Ross HM: Societal/cultural views regarding death and dying, *Top Clin Nurs* 1(1):1, 1981.

◆ YUGOSLAVIA (BOSNIA-HERZEGOVINA)

MAP PAGE (258)

Location: The former Yugoslavia is located in southeast Europe on the Balkan Peninsula along the Adriatic Sea and consists of Serbia and Montenegro, Bosnia-Herzegovina, Croatia-Slavonia, and Dalmatia. At this time Serbia is the only geographic area to which the name Yugoslavia applies.

Major Languages	Ethnic Groups		Major Religions	
Serbo-Croatian	Serb	36%	Greek	
Slovene	Croat	20%	Orthodox	50%
Macedonian	Muslim	9%	Catholic	30%
Albanian	Slovene	8%	Muslim	10%
Hungarian	Albanian		Other	10%
	and Other	27%		

Ethnic/Race Specific or Endemic Diseases: RISK: Coronary heart disease; colon cancer; adult onset insulin-dependent diabetes.

National Childhood Immunizations: BCG at birth; DPT at 3 months, 4½ months, 6 months, 18 months, and 3½ years; DT at 7 years and at 14 years; OPV at 3 months, 4½ months, 6 months, 18 months, 3½ years, 7 years, and 14 years; MMR at 16 months in 3 republics and MM in one republic; measles at 16 months but not until 7 years in one republic; rubella for girls at 13 years in 3 republics.

BIBLIOGRAPHY

Aspell T: NBC News, June 15, 1992.

Benson ER: The legend of the Maiden of Kosovo and nursing in Serbia, *Image* 23(1):57, 1991.

Brokaw T: NBC News, June 25, 1991.

Reeser DS: An international experience, *Imprint* 32(1):46, 1985.

Solomon J: Critical care nursing, *Focus Crit Care* 13(3):10, 1986.

◆ ZAIRE

MAP PAGE (261)

Location: Formerly the Belgian Congo, Zaire is located around the equator in central Africa with one small arm extending west and providing a short strip of Atlantic Ocean coastline. The Zaire (Congo) River traverses the land. The terrain includes low plateaus covered with a rain forest and grasslands, and high mountains are in the east.

Major Languages	Ethnic Groups		Major Religions	
French	Bantu Groups	80%	Catholic	50%
English	Other	20%	Protestant	20%
Lingala			Kimbanguist	10%
Swahili			Muslim	10%
Kikongo			Other	10%
and Other				

Ethnic/Race Specific or Endemic Diseases: ACTIVE: Cholera; yellow fever. ENDEMIC: Chloroquine-resistant malaria. RISK: Schistosomiasis.

National Childhood Immunizations: BCG at birth; DPT-1 at 6 weeks; DPT-2 at 10 weeks; DPT-3 at 14 weeks; measles at 9 months; OPV at birth; OPV-1 at 6 weeks; OPV-2 at 10 weeks; OPV-3 at 14 weeks.

BIBLIOGRAPHY
No data located.

◆ ZAMBIA

MAP PAGE (261)

Location: This landlocked republic (formerly Northern Rhodesia) is located in south Africa and consists of high, forested plateaus drained by large rivers. The climate is subtropical, and the country is subject to drought and famine.

Major Languages	Ethnic Groups		Major Religions	
English	African	99%	Christian	65%
African	European		Indigenous	
Languages	and Other	1%	Beliefs	34%
			Muslim	
			and Hindu	1%

Ethnic/Race Specific or Endemic Diseases: ACTIVE: Cholera. **ENDEMIC:** Yellow fever; chloroquine-resistant malaria. **RISK:** Schistosomiasis. AIDS case rate is 16.5/ 100,000 people.

National Childhood Immunizations: BCG at birth; DPT-1 at 2 months; DPT-2 at 3 months; DPT-3 at 4 months; measles at 8 months; OPV-1 at 2 months; OPV-2 at 3 months; OPV-3 at 4 months.

BIBLIOGRAPHY

Adler MW, editor: Statistics from the World Health Organization and the Centers for Disease Control, *AIDS* 6(10):1229, 1992.
Pauley J: NBC News, June 22, 1992.

◆ ZIMBABWE

MAP PAGE (261)

Location: This landlocked south-central African country (formerly Southern Rhodesia) has high plateaus and mountains in the east. The climate is subtropical. Most people live in small villages and are engaged in subsistence farming.

Major Languages	Ethnic Groups		Major Religions	
English	Shona	71%	Syncretic	50%
Chishona	Ndebele	16%	Christian	25%
Sindebele	White	1%	Indigenous Beliefs	24%
	Other	12%	Muslim	1%

Ethnic/Race Specific or Endemic Diseases: ENDEMIC: Chloroquine-resistant malaria. RISK: Schistosomiasis. AIDS case rate is 44.9/100,000 people.

National Childhood Immunizations: BCG at birth; DPT-1 at 3 months; DPT-2 at 4 months; DPT-3 at 5 months; DPT booster at 18 months; OPV plus DT plus BCG at 5 years; measles at 9 months; OPV-1 at 3 months; OPV-2 at 4 months; OPV-3 at 5 months; OPV booster at 18 months.

BIBLIOGRAPHY

Adler MW, editor: Statistics from the World Health Organization and the Centers for Disease Control, *AIDS* 6(10):1229, 1992.

Utley G: Report of the Amsterdam Conference on AIDS, NBC News, July 18, 1992.

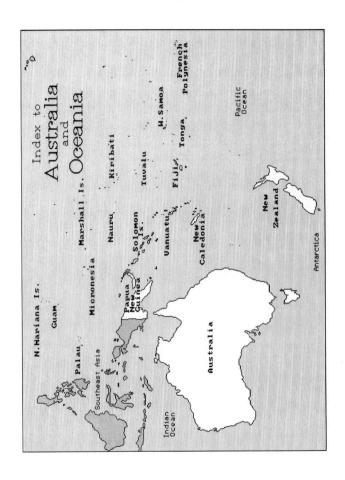

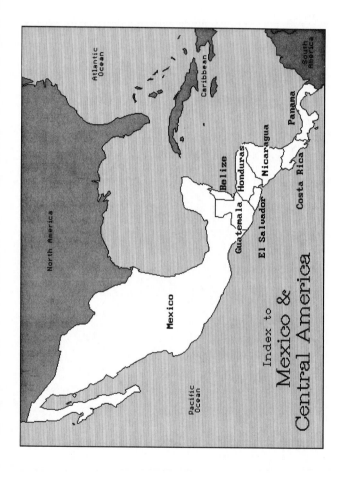

Index to
Mexico &
Central America

North America

Atlantic
Ocean

Caribbean

South
America

Panama

Belize

Honduras

Nicaragua

Guatemala

El Salvador

Costa Rica

Mexico

Pacific
Ocean

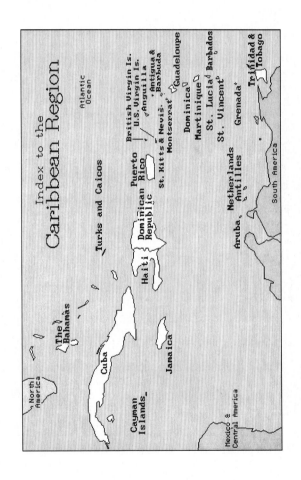

Index to the
Caribbean Region

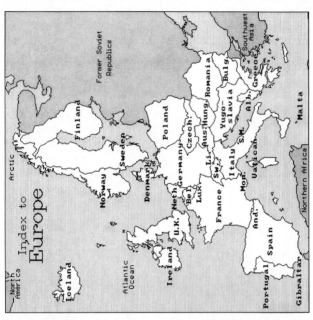

Index to Europe

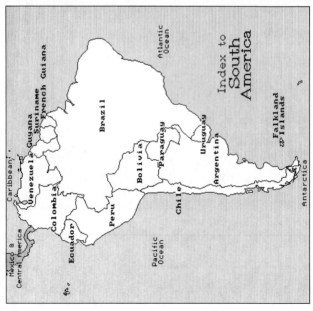

Index to South America

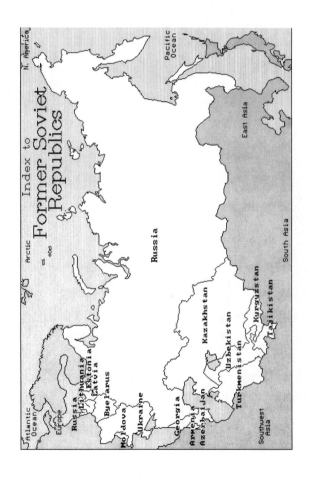

Index to Former Soviet Republics

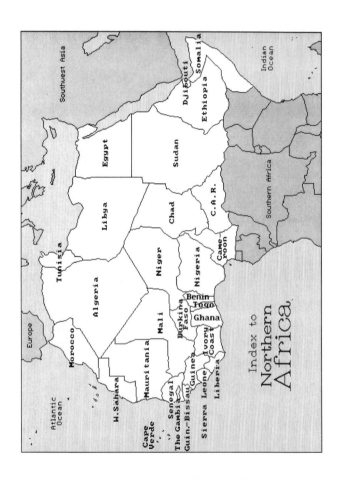

Index to Northern Africa

Europe

Atlantic Ocean

Southwest Asia

Indian Ocean

Southern Africa

Morocco

W.Sahara

Mauritania

Cape Verde

Senegal

The Gambia

Guin.-Bissau

Guinea

Sierra Leone

Liberia

Ivory Coast

Ghana

Togo

Benin

Burkina Faso

Mali

Algeria

Tunisia

Libya

Niger

Nigeria

Cameroon

Chad

C.A.R.

Egypt

Sudan

Ethiopia

Djibouti

Somalia

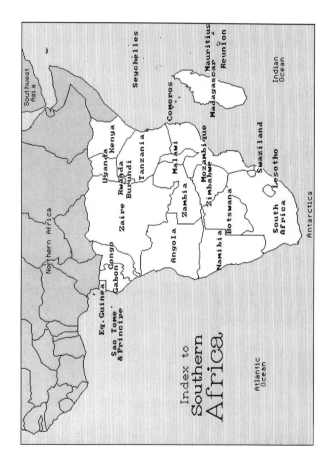

Index to
Southern Africa

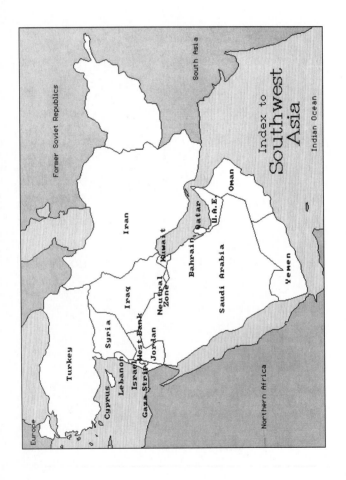

Index to
Southwest
Asia

Former Soviet Republics

South Asia

Indian Ocean

Europe

Turkey

Cyprus

Lebanon

Syria

Iran

Israel

West Bank

Gaza Strip

Jordan

Iraq

Neutral Zone

Kuwait

Bahrain

Qatar

U.A.E.

Oman

Saudi Arabia

Yemen

Northern Africa

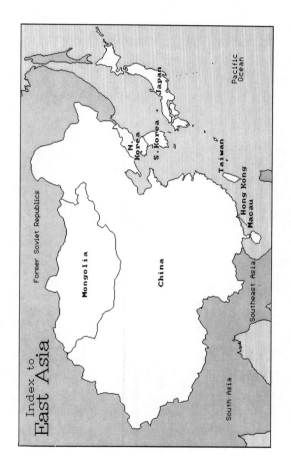

Index to
East Asia

Former Soviet Republics

Mongolia

China

N. Korea

S. Korea

Japan

Taiwan

Hong Kong

Macau

Pacific Ocean

Southeast Asia

South Asia

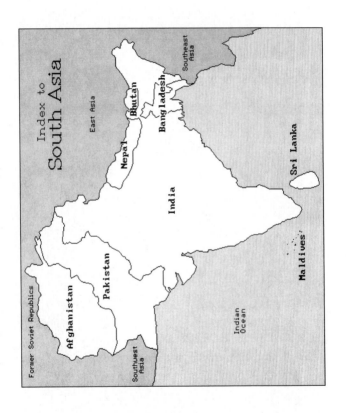

Index to South Asia

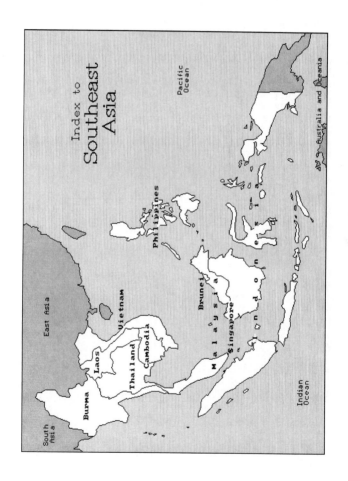

Index to
Southeast
Asia

East Asia

South
Asia

Burma

Laos

Thailand

Vietnam

Cambodia

Philippines

Brunei

M a l a y s i a

Singapore

I n d o n e s i a

Pacific
Ocean

Indian
Ocean

Australia and Oceania

Ethnic group index